'Does Speech and Language Therapy Work?' A Review of the Literature

'Does Speech and Language Therapy Work?'

A Review of the Literature

Pam Enderby and Joyce Emerson
Speech and Language Therapy Research Unit
Frenchay Hospital
Bristol BS16 1LE

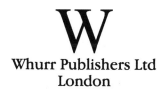

Whurr Publishers Ltd
London

© 1995 Whurr Publishers
First published 1995 by
Whurr Publishers Ltd
19b Compton Terrace, London N1 2UN, England

Reprinted 1996

British Library Cataloguing in Publication Data
A catalogue record for this book is available from the
British Library.

ISBN 1-897635-38-9

Printed and bound in the UK by Athenaeum Press Ltd, Gateshead,
Tyne & Wear

Contents

Acknowledgements

Many specialist advisers to the College of Speech and Language Therapists have assisted by providing and tracking down references as well as commenting on drafts of chapters related to their areas of interest. We thank them all for their prompting, suggestions and goading.

This work was commissioned by the Department of Health. We thank them for their interest in the field and their support and encouragement.

The views expressed in this book are those of the authors and not necessarily of the Department of Health

Note to Readers

It is expected that readers may wish to dwell particularly on the chapter or chapters related to the client group that is of particular interest to them. It is suggested that the reader puts the chapter in context by also reading the introduction and conclusion which will assist with interpretation.

Chapter 1
Introduction

Purpose

The purpose of this study was to review the international literature in order to establish the state of knowledge regarding the efficacy of speech and language therapy with the major client groups, and to identify key areas for future research investment. This required the identification of the most significant published research carried out referring to speech and language treatment methods and related studies of efficacy leading to a critical analysis. Whilst this purpose appears to be clear the work presented here is broader than originally intended. The importance of setting efficacy literature in a context in order to establish its relevance and validity, and to assist with interpretation cannot be underestimated. For example, we have found it important to review information regarding prevalence of different speech and language disorders in order to inform the priorities for future research. Furthermore, speech and language therapy research can rarely be undertaken in isolation of research in related disciplines. Thus, the efficacy of speech and language therapy in many fields is closely related to the knowledge and principles related to the treatment of the underlying causes or associated difficulties.

Research and the NHS

Research connected to efficacy of speech and language therapy is desirable in order that therapists may offer an improved quality of life, as effectively as possible, to the maximum number of people. It has been generally recognized that much treatment within the health service has been based upon history and anecdote. Current changes in the health-care system are necessitating more evidence of knowledge-based practice to underpin service delivery and development. It has become axiomatic that clinical practice should be based on research evidence (Doehring, 1988; Hedge, 1987; Silverman, 1977; Ventry and Schiavetti, 1980). The importance of literature reviews to anchor evidence-based

provision is becoming increasingly common (Haines and Jones, 1994).
Thus, many health commissioners are currently seeking pertinent critical appraisal of the literature in order to inform their decision making. A
necessary dialogue between those who know the questions, the health-
care provider and purchaser, and those who can assist with the answers
(researchers), is developing – and not before time. 'The objective of the
NHS R&D Strategy is to ensure that the content and delivery of care in
the NHS is based on high quality research relevant to improving the
health of the nation' (Research for Health, 1991). In order to achieve this
it is important to identify the priority areas requiring attention.

Literature Reviews

Literature reviews are always problematic, most reviewers put in considerable efforts, but the results are almost inevitably variable (Mulrow,
1987) as there are a few accepted standards to ensure that literature
reviews are comprehensive and balanced (Powe *et al.*, 1994). Not all the
recommended practices have been able to be used within this document. For example, if we had taken the systematic approach recommended by the Cochrane collaboration (Oxman, 1994) the review
would have been too short to enable identification of priorities within
the necessary context. Some reviews have limited themselves to certain
styles of evaluation. However, we have not, as not only have there been
few controlled trials within speech and language therapy, but also this
type of research alone is not appropriate to this speciality, giving a false
impression of the knowledge base. A range of other methodologies not
traditionally used within the medical field but more commonly associated with social science and education, have been appropriately used to
clarify some domains and are therefore included.

Similar to other literature reviews, we have found that, 'for every bit
of research that comes to any specific conclusion, there is at least one
research report that disagrees' (Sommers, Logsdon and Wright 1992).
Literature reviews that aim to organize and compile findings are
frequently open to criticism for including some studies, which may be
viewed as inappropriate or weak, for making subjective conclusions or
for excluding or omitting other research for whatever reason. It is hard
to collate information without an element of subjectivity and personal
bias, which may aim to illuminate, but in fact can cloud an issue.

This review struggled for a coherent approach to give a common
format for each chapter. The disparity in the way that different specialist
areas have been approached, the varying emphasis on topic areas and
the difference in volume of relevant research or underlying literature
made this difficult. Reviews, after all, can only reflect and display what
has been done and a lack of coherence between topic areas is, in itself, of
interest in considering priorities. We are conscious in our review that we

have drawn heavily on American literature. Whilst this reflects the greater investment in research in that country and the longer history of relevant postgraduate education, we are concerned that there are professional, educational, political and healthcare funding factors that should caution blanket adoption of results. Furthermore, whilst searching the grey literature to some extent, we have depended mostly on published literature, which may lead to a certain bias as positive and significant results are more likely to be accepted (Oxman and Guyatt 1988).

The following questions relating to the efficacy of speech rehabilitation were proposed by Darley (1972):

- Does speech and language therapy accomplish measurable gains – does therapy have an influence on the course of the recovery?
- Are the gains worth the necessary investment in time, effort and money?
- What are the relative degrees of effectiveness of various modes of therapy?

These questions have more recently been updated. Bain and Dollaghan (1991) in their contribution to a review on recent research emphasize the importance of clinically significant change, which they suggest contains three dimensions:

- to result from treatment rather than from maturation or other uncontrolled factors;
- to be real rather than random;
- to be important rather than trivial.

Previous literature reviews related to the communication area by Bloch and Goodstein (1971), Sommers *et al.* (1979) and Bryen and Joyce (1985) have all highlighted concerns related to:

- weaknesses in subject classification criteria that place major restrictions upon the generalization of research findings;
- the absence of, or limited use of, reliability and validity measures;
- the lack of empirical cause/effect data to support the conclusion drawn;
- lack of control groups, inappropriate or no randomization techniques and generally weak research designs.

Since these reviews, there has been development in the knowledge regarding the difficulties related to studies in this field and acknowledgement that traditional research designs may be inappropriate for some topics.

A more recent review by Sommers, Logsdon and Wright (1992) concludes that patterns in the literature were found that corresponded to the changes in theory and practice over the two decades 'although some positive changes occurred, negative research practices continued from the 1970s into the 1980s' they identified common difficulties with interpreting the literature as follows; lack of subject detail, lack of research related to client groups that predominate in the clinics, i.e. those with compound and complex difficulties, lack of detail with regard to the type and quality of treatment, lack of random selection and inadequate sample sizes in quantitative studies. They note that recently there was an increase in the number of single subject design studies reported and a decline in the 1980s of large group studies. Remarking on this latter occurrence, the authors quite rightly note that single subject designs have made substantial contributions to the testing of experimental hypotheses involving treatment but it is regrettable that replications of single subject findings, using larger numbers of subjects from the same population, are not appearing in the literature.

Research Designs

Randomized control trials (RCTs) are believed, in medicine (Cochrane 1972), to be the most powerful evidence of the effects of treatment. Whilst there are various forms of random control trial, in essence the subjects are randomly assigned to either a treatment group, which receives the prescribed therapy, or to the control group, which receives attention of some kind. The results are compared by assessors who may be 'blind', i.e. have no knowledge of which group the patient comes from.

RCTs have been carried out in investigations of the efficacy of speech and language therapy notably in studies of aphasia. However, this type of study has been one which therapists have criticized on the grounds that: it is not ethically defensible to withhold treatment that is believed to be effective; it is hard to match heterogenous groups; and it is difficult to maintain the 'blindness' of assessors. It has been suggested that treatment groups should be compared with a group where treatment is unavailable, or that control groups should receive the prescribed treatment at a later stage. Attempts such as these, to get around ethical problems, might add to methodological weaknesses regarding homogeneity of population and consistency of treatment. A further objection to RCTs, as a means of assessing the effectiveness of speech and language therapy, is that speech and language impaired populations are not homogenous groups. The impact of variations, such as aetiological variations, age, gender, educational background and psychosocial factors, may have bearings on the outcome to treatment but are difficult to control in randomization except by stratification, which requires a considerably greater number of subjects and therefore may be difficult to recruit if the disorder is of low incidence or the research resources are limited. Furthermore, the therapy received cannot be regarded as 'one treatment' in the same way as a drug treatment because therapists work in different ways from each other and apply varying treatments to their different subjects. The idea that variations in the relationship between the patient and the therapist may have a bearing on the outcome of treatment further complicates the use of RCTs (Howard 1986; Pring 1989).

The single case experimental design has been advocated as the most appropriate design for the study of efficacy of speech and language therapy with aphasic individuals (Pring 1989) and is widely used in other fields. By varying aspects, such as the time treatment commenced, or the type of treatment given, it may be possible to identify change on particular tasks or items, as being due to specific techniques of therapy, rather than the effects of treatment in general, or of external factors such as spontaneous recovery. This type of study, though taking time to prepare and analyse, may be easier to undertake as it is less disruptive to clinical practice and offers advantages over the most frequent account of treatment in the literature, the case study, which can be of limited use in providing evidence for the effectiveness of treatments since there can be no account taken of extrinsic factors which may contribute to the patient's improvement. However, there are problems with single case studies. Many of those reported give exemplary detail regarding the treatment progress, but little information on the subject, thereby making it hard to generalize. Furthermore, there are few single case studies submitted for publication/or published that have negative results. It is essential that single case studies are replicated to establish the claims that are based on the evidence of one individual.

In a monograph entitled 'The future of science and services', Goldstein (1990) passes on a maxim from the applied behaviour analysis folklore 'arguing that it takes three studies on one intervention before really meaningful results are revealed. Scientists who demonstrate such persistence find it difficult to argue with this rule of thumb.' This maxim is consistent with the obligation of scientists to guard against premature dissemination of research lacking adequate empirical support.

Muma (1993) stresses the need for replication in order to provide verification and disconfirmation. As many studies of the efficacy of speech and language therapy have small sample sizes, or use single case design, replication would be helpful in reducing the chances of false findings, and would extend the possibility of generalization. Muma notes that a minority of speech and language studies are attempts at replication, which may be related to the replication being of little interest to researchers or the funders of research

Meta-analysis, a quantitative approach that examines a series of group studies, usually of the random control type, and summarizes the findings, has been used in speech and language therapy research to examine the efficacy of stroke treatment (Whurr *et al.*, 1992). Guidelines in the use of meta-analysis in evaluating experimental studies and interpretation of the results have been suggested (Sacks *et al.*, 1987; L'Abbé *et al.*, 1987) and stress the importance of a comprehensive literature search, consideration of variations in individuals studies, the need to reduce the possibility of bias, and the use of sensitive techniques for pooling results. Meta-analysis has been criticized in trying to pool studies which have subtly different client groups, different treatment emphasis, and use different outcome measures. There is a strong possibility that by adding apples and pears one will end up with a fruit salad of results that may bear little relationship to the original ingredients. Meta-analysis, which is being primarily used to evaluate the results of various medical and surgical investigations, requires some adaptation for its use within other scientific areas.

Some practitioners (e.g. Eastwood, 1988) have advocated the adoption of a qualitative methodology for the investigation of speech and language therapy. In qualitative research the investigator acknowledges the part that investigation plays in the study and conducts careful observation by means of participation in, or observation of, activity, or by unstructured questionnaires. This method allows the development of theories rather than the testing of established theories as does the quantitative methodology. Hoit (1990) surveyed 21 well known speech and language therapy researchers in the United States of America and elicited that many felt that 'the important missing element of our knowledge as still descriptive. Our field skipped over the pre-science age, the descriptive age, and has tried to be theoretical and experimental, prematurely and possibly incorrectly.' In contrast, some other well-known researchers put forward the view that the research should be more theory driven and they express concern that the field is 'stuck in the descriptive stage'; this dichotomy is probably related to the disciplines and interests of the researchers. Our review indicates that some studies have a good basis of description allowing firm underpinning for hypothesis testing. Other areas have not achieved that status.

Quantitative and qualitative approaches should be complementary. Good, well observed qualitative studies can lead to the development of theories that can then be tested using quantitative methods: the results of quantitative studies may lead to a search for reasons for the results which may fuel qualitative studies. In practice, the two approaches seem to be in conflict. Qualitative studies, as so described, have made little impact on the literature under consideration, apart from the single case studies which often use some qualitative methods such as description.

Recent research studies have reflected the increasing concern that a successful outcome of therapy should be seen in terms of the impact on communication in everyday life and its overall impact on the client (Bain and Dollaghan, 1991; Enderby, 1992). Changes in functional communication are frequently used as a criterion for the efficacy of treatment. Methods of capturing changes in conversation, social interaction and general communication are more difficult than traditional sound analysis and word counts. Thus, the philosophy that researchers must consider the impact of therapy more holistically has necessitated either the use of poorly developed tools to capture this difficult area, or the expenditure of time on developing more appropriate assessment tools, which hopefully will be of assistance in the future. Research can only be seen in the broader context of society and its politics. More recently, both language tests and approaches to treatment are being challenged as being 'disablement based' rather than centred on the individual. New approaches, aimed to place more emphasis on defects in society that marginalize people with impairments leading normal lives, are being called for (Barnes, 1992).

Changes in the health service delivery have placed more emphasis on the financial implications of providing treatments. Speech and language therapists, along with all other health service staff, are under pressure to prove the efficiency and effectiveness of their work in order to inform purchasing and delivery decisions. The constraints under which therapists work can act as an incentive to find more effective ways of treatment to match resources. The impact of variations in ways that service is financed is clear throughout the literature, including that from the United States of America where issues such as whether the patient is paying for treatment influence the aims and conduct of research.

The profession is currently coming to terms with the problems posed by the definition of what constitutes a successful outcome for all groups of people with which the profession is involved (van der Gaag, 1993). Attempts are being made to define the outcome of therapy in ways which are intelligible, coherent for therapists to use and for others to understand. The importance of incorporating patients' and relatives' views in goal setting and judgements of benefits have been called for for some time (Light and Pillemer, 1984; Enderby, 1992).

Methodology of this Literature Review

The diversity of the professional activities of speech and language therapists with the many different client groups that have communication disorders is reflected in the number of journals which publish related papers on communication, science and disorders. Speech and language therapists publish work within specialist journals, medical and surgical journals, and in journals which cover linguistics, education, psychology, behavioral sciences, engineering, etc. In a review of journals primarily reporting communication science, and disorder literature, Jackson and Hale report 67 journals (Jackson and Hale, 1990). Thus, a search of various computer data-bases was necessary for each specialty in order to capture the most recent and relevant research. The following data-bases were used in this search:

- Medline
- Embase Psychiatry
- Cumulative Index to Nursing and Allied Health (CINAHL)
- Psych-Info
- Language and Linguistics Behavioral Abstracts (LLBA)
- Frenchay Speech and Language Therapy.

In addition, all of the College of Speech and Language Therapist Special Advisors, in the specific clinical areas, were contacted and asked for a list of significant references on treatment efficacy in their specialist field. Recently published and the most frequently used text books were consulted for background and general information relating to the topics.

The grey literature was searched by contacting the English Universities/Colleges, where speech and language therapists, under-graduates and post-graduates are trained, in order to inspect the titles of post-graduate dissertations. This did not elicit a very significant amount of information related to efficacy. The preliminary drafts of each chapter were sent to three specialist speech and language therapists, mostly CSLT advisors. Their comments and additional recommended literature were considered and incorporated in this final presentation.

There was little literature on the efficacy of speech and language therapy related to some client groups, e.g. mental health, dysphagia and hearing impairment – this is probably due to the relative recency of SLT being involved in the managment of these disorders. Thus the review is confined to acquired dysphasia, children with speech and language disorders, cleft palate, dysarthria, laryngectomy, learning disabilities, stammering and voice disorders.

References

Bain BA and Dollaghan CA (1991). The notion of clinically significant change: Treatment efficacy. Language, Speech and Hearing Services in Schools 22: 264–270.

Barnes C (1992). Qualitative research: Valuable or irrelevant? Disability Handicap and Society 7(2): 115–124.

Bloch EL and Goodstein LD (1971). Functional speech disorders and personality: A decade of research. Journal of Speech and Hearing Disorders 36: 295–314.

Bryen DN and Joyce DG (1985). Language intervention with the severely handicapped: A decade of research. The Journal of Special Education 19(1): 7–39.

Cochrane AL (1972). Effectiveness and Efficiency: Random Reflections on Health Services. London: Nuffield Provincial Hospital Trust.

Darley FL (1972). The efficacy of language rehabilitation in aphasia. Journal of Speech and Hearing Disorders 37: 3–21.

Doehring DG (1988). Research Strategies in Human Communication Disorders. Boston, MA: Little, Brown, 4–6.

Eastwood J (1988). Qualitative research: An additional research methodology for speech pathology? British Journal of Disorders of Communication 23(2): 71–184.

Enderby P (1992). Outcome measures in speech therapy: Impairment, disability, handicap and distress. Health Trends 24(2): 61–64.

Goldstein H (1990). The future of language science: A plea for language intervention research. The Future of Science and Services Seminar. ASHA Reports Number 20: 41–50.

Haines A and Jones R (1994). Implementing findings of research. British Medical Journal 308: 1488–1492.

Hedge MN (1987). Clinical Research in Communicative Disorders: Principles and Strategies. Boston, MA: College Hill Press.

Hoit JD (1990). Peering into the future. The future of science and services seminar. ASHA Reports Number 20: 61–68.

Howard D (1986). Beyond randomised controlled trials: The case for effective case studies of the effect of treatment in aphasia. British Journal of Disorders of Communication 21: 89–102.

Jackson PD and Hale ST (1990). Journal in Communication Sciences and Disorders: A Resource Guide for Authors. Rockville, MD: American Speech and Language Hearing Association.

L'Abbé KA, Detsky AS and O'Rourke K (1987). Meta-analysis in clinical research. Annals of Internal Medicine 107: 224–233.

Light RJ and Pillemer DB (1984). Summing Up: The Science of Reviewing Research. Cambridge, MA: Harvard University Press, 3, 4.

Mulrow CD (1987). The medical review article: State of the science. Ann; Int; Med 106: 485–488.

Muma JR (1993). The need for replication. Journal of Speech and Hearing Research 36: 927–930.

Oxman A (Ed) (1994). Preparing and Maintaining Systematic Reviews. Cochrane Collaboration Handbook 1994. VI–1. Oxford: Cochrane Collaboration.

Oxman AD and Guyatt GH (1988). Guidelines for reading literature reviews. The Canadian Medical Association Journal 138: 697–703.

Powe NR, Turner JA, Maklan CW and Erzek M (1994). Alternative methods for formal literature review and meta-analysis in AHCPR patient outcomes research teams. Agency for Medical Care Policy and Research 32(7 suppl): 22–37.

Pring TR (1989). Evaluating the effects of speech therapy for aphasics and volunteers: Developing the single case methodology. British Journal of Disorder of Communication 21: 103–115.

Research for Health: Research and Development Strategy for the NHS (1991). London: HMSO Department of Health.

Sacks HS, Berrier J, Reitman D, Ancona-Berk VA and Chalmers TC (1987). Meta-Analysis of randomized controlled trials. New England Journal of Medicine 316(8): 450–454.

Silverman FH (1977). Research Design in Speech Pathology and Audiology. Englewood Cliffs, NY: Prentice Hall.

Sommers RK, Bobkoff-Leventhal K, Applegate JA and Square PA (1979). A critical review of a recent decade of stuttering research. Journal of Fluency Disorders 4: 223–237.

Sommers RK, Logsdon BS and Wright JM (1992). A review and critical analysis of treatment research related to articulation and phonological disorders. Journal of Communication Disorders 25: 3–22.

van der Gaag A (1993). Outcome Research in Speech and Language Therapy. Audit: a manual for speech and language therapists. London: College of Speech and Language Therapists.

Ventry IM and Schiavetti N (1980). Evaluating Research in Speech Pathology and Audiology: (2nd Edition). New York: MacMillan.

Whurr R, Lorch MP and Nye C (1992). A meta-analysis of studies carried out between 1946 and 1988 concerned with the efficacy of speech and language therapy treatment for aphasic patients. European Journal of Disorders of Communication 27(1): 1–17.

Chapter 2
Acquired Dysphasia

Introduction

Dysphasia[1] can be the result of, commonly, a stroke, or less commonly, a head injury and is defined as a defect or loss of the power of expression by speech, writing or gesture, as well as that of comprehending spoken or written language. This definition rightly suggests a spectrum of disorders of both expression and comprehension that are attributable to cerebral dysfunction. Although the term dysphasia refers to a lesser degree of severity of the same problem as aphasia, these terms are frequently used interchangeably. Of the 220 persons per 100 000 population who have a first or a recurrent stroke each year, approximately 66 will have this language disorder. The prevalence of persisting speech and language disorder at 6 months following a stroke would be a further 50 per 100 000 (Enderby and Davies, 1989). The effects of dysphasia on the individual, the family and society are numerous and significant. Determining the best rehabilitation programmes to restore communication skills to these individuals has challenged the research community for many decades.

The papers reviewed here address the many issues that may affect the recovery of dysphasia. It has been suggested that age, sex; site, size and type of lesion; personality, literacy levels, educational attainment, psychological make-up, and social circumstances as well as speech and language therapy can be seen as possibly influencing outcome.

Age of onset is thought to affect the outcome for the aphasic patient in that younger patients recover better or at least the prognosis for recovery is better (Keenan and Brassell 1974; Sarno *et al.*, 1970). The Shewan and Kertesz (1984) study confirmed this.

There seems to be a higher frequency of aphasia in male than in female patients, approximately 3:1, but this may reflect referral bias. However, gender does not seem to be related to recovery – both male and female subjects performing similarly in most studies.

[1]In this document the terms aphasia and dysphasia are used interchangeably

11

Therapy

It is beyond the scope of this document to describe the many therapeutic approaches that have been developed to assist dysphasic individuals, but the significant themes that have evolved will be summarized briefly. Therapy tends to polarize from one of general language stimulation or general language encouragement to that of domain specific treatment (Lyon, 1992). Along with these two approaches has been a trend towards more emphasis on counselling to assist with psychosocial adjustment and the employment of techniques to facilitate both verbal and non-verbal communication skills.

Schuell, Jenkins and Jiminez-Pabon (1964) postulated that therapy does not aim to teach new material to the patient but rather to maximize the efficiency of an impaired language system. In Schuell's general stimulation therapy, the clinician supplied a variety of auditory and visual models and cues to elicit responses from the patient. This approach is based on the hypothesis that word-retrieval processes can be stimulated generally. Despite the widespread use of Schuell's stimulation approach, many authors have reservations regarding the theoretical base and additionally point to the major limitation that the approach does not consider the functional context of communication and tends to advocate a blanket approach to all different aphasic deficits.

To address functional use of language or language in context Davis and Wilcox (1985) proposed a procedure termed PACE (promoting aphasics' communicative effectiveness) which reshapes therapy into a form more closely resembling face-to-face conversation. In this approach the client and clinician engage in a sequence of interactions, alternating turns as senders and receivers of the message. The message should be unknown to the receiver. In addition, patients are encouraged to use multiple channels, including gestures, to communicate.

A number of different approaches have been employed for treating a specific dysphasic deficit termed anomia. Some therapies, such as BASE-10 Programmed Stimulation, have emphasized a relearning approach (La Pointe, 1977). Specialized stimuli (vocabulary – usually nouns) are chosen and practised until a predetermined criterion level is reached. The next group of words are then identified and practised.

This description has already fallen into the trap, identified by Byng (1993), of the serious gap in therapy literature:

> What a clinician does becomes somehow intrinsic to his, or her, performance. There seems to be a kind of 'automatic pilot' that a good clinician develops and then switches on which suggests how to present a task, how and when to modulate it, how to respond to a specific response by a specific patient, and so on . . . Most accounts of therapy take seriously only the role of the therapist

and the task and materials. The impact of how the patient responds to what the therapist does is not described; therapists proceed in therapy by modifying the task, their manner of responding, or what they ask the patient to do . . .

The discipline of neuro-psycholinguistics has influenced the study of aphasia over many decades. The roots of these theories originated in the treatise by Freund (1889) which has recently been translated by Beaton, Davidoff and Erstfeld (1991). The main hypothesis is that language is represented by a connective network of modality-specific systems. Interactive modules and language sub-strata systems have been postulated to assist in explaining the underlying structure of language and its relationship to meaning. One reason that these had been developed was in order to refine the classifications and definitions of aphasic syndromes and to simplify the diverse combination of language deficits. Neurolinguistic approaches allow hypotheses for the underlying deficit to be made explicit, and therefore used to guide therapy. Previous approaches had relied on surface symptomatology as a basis for the description of the disorder and for determining therapy.

Different modes of therapy delivery have also been considered over the last 20 years. These include the use of untrained volunteers, telephone therapy and group delivery. In addition, computerized therapy is now attracting attention. The micro-computer's ability to perform repetitive tasks with endless patience, together with its facility for the provision of immediate and dynamic feedback, indicates that it may suit the dysphasic patient extremely well.

This extremely brief review of the nature of therapy does not do justice to the extensive literature in this field.

Efficacy

There have been more studies into the efficacy of speech and language therapy for dysphasia, published over the past two decades, than for any other client group. However, it is still difficult to answer categorically the question of whether speech and language therapy 'works', also what 'works' means, i.e. what constitutes a positive outcome has yet to be defined. Therapy may aim to enhance existing language skills, teach new ones, assist psychological adjustments, enable carers to communicate successfully, etc. All these different aspects of therapy have not been evaluated for their effectiveness (Byng, 1993). Therefore, studies carried out do not reflect what therapists do. It is difficult to combine the results of these studies, as the methodologies adopted, the aetiologies of the patients, the types and severities of aphasia represented, and the nature of treatment, have differed widely.

Many studies have not given specific information about all these areas. The problem is confounded by the different underlying philosophies of the speech and language therapy, and its change of perspective over the last 20 years following a radical evolution of the understanding of the nature of the deficit of aphasia.

Group studies

Many of the early studies were documentary in nature indicating the effects of treatment and the recovery of aphasia in general ways (Godfrey and Douglass, 1959; Marks *et al.*, 1957). These historically interesting studies show a maturity in investigation and enquiry but a naivety in methodology; for example, Butfield and Zangwill (1946), investigated the effect of treatment on a group of 70 aphasic patients. Fourteen had head injuries, 19 had had a stroke (vascular aetiology), and 37 had neoplastic lesions. The patients were divided into two groups, those whose therapy began less than 6 months after onset of aphasia and those whose therapy began more than 6 months after onset. All patients received treatment. Speech improved in more than half of the first group and nearly one-third of the second, but the mixed aetiologies of the patients preclude firm inferences being drawn.

Mixed aetiologies confounded another early study (Marks *et al.*, 1957), which reported the results of a follow-up study of 324 patients aged between 30 and 60 years. Aphasia was caused by CVA in 190 patients and traumatic injuries in 13 patients. There is no indication as to the cause of aphasia in the remaining 121 patients. The patients conditions were categorized as expressive, receptive, mixed or global. On initial examination, 97 of the patients had both aphasic and dysarthric symptoms. Forty of the patients received no therapy. Evaluation of the patients was based on a subjective four-point scale. The resulting recovery was classified as excellent in 6.9% of the patients, good in 22%, fair in 21% and poor in 49%. Despite some aspects being detailed it is still difficult to interpret this study as, supposedly, 324 patients were studied, but only 198 patients were accounted for in discharge follow-up and only 129 are accounted for in the results. Furthermore, 40 patients were listed as having no therapy while in-patients, and 102 as having no therapy after discharge but these individuals are not accounted for in the statistics.

It was not until much later that controls for the type of treatment, treatment versus no treatment, and the amount of treatment were considered as necessary variables. For example, Vignolo (1964) addressed the efficacy question more rigorously, reporting a retrospective clinical study with both treated and control groups. While the overall difference between the two groups was not statistically significant, the data suggested that treatment was generally efficacious, particularly if it was initiated early (prior to 6 months post onset of aphasia) and if continued for a substantial period 'at least 6 months'. Subsequent reports with an expanded population claim to have statistically confirmed these positive effects of rehabilitation (Basso *et al.*, 1979).

The control groups in these studies were not randomly assigned and the criticism could be made that this permitted selection variables to operate which may have biased the control to include poorer candidates for recovery. Basso and her co-workers, concerned about this possibility, examined records and reported that the selection variables for the untreated group were not related to aphasia and, although they were older, age was not found to be a factor affecting outcome.

In the few studies that have used matched control groups, the results have been conflicting regarding the efficacy of treatment. Hagen (1973) compared 10 patients sequentially allocated to an intensive therapy group with 10 patients in a no-treatment group. The author reported significantly greater improvement in the treated group particularly in comprehension, language formulation, speech production, spelling and arithmetic. Whilst the subjects were a single type (Schuells Group III), there was no control for the severity of aphasia. He concluded that some spontaneous remission accounts for recovery of some aspects such as visual comprehension, auditory comprehension and auditory retention abilities. 'Speech production and reading comprehension ability spontaneously improved during the first 6 months post onset but not to a functional level';

> 'It may well be that treatment is a process of channelling spontaneous recovery and compensating for deficits. Since the greatest gains in spontaneous recovery seem to occur during the first 6 months after stroke, it may be that the earlier treatment is initiated, the greater will be the results over time. On the other hand, the subjects in the treatment group benefit from treatment initiated 6 months post onset' (Hagen, 1973).

Some of the speculation and discussion about this argument, whilst stimulating, is not supported by the data and the findings.

The study by Sarno, Silverman and Sands (1970) did not corroborate Hagen's findings as their aphasics did not improve, regardless of the type of treatment or whether they received treatment at all. The study by Sarno is another historical landmark; it compared two types of treatment, programmed learning and non-programmed learning, and a no-treatment group. This study included only severe (global) aphasics. Since this study was conducted there has been evidence that the severity of aphasia is generally considered to influence recovery outcome, such that severe aphasics start with the lowest scores and improve the least. In view of this it is impossible to generalize the results of either to the overall aphasic population.

A study, with improved design and methodology, by Shewan and Kertesz (1984) recruited 100 patients, sequentially referred, and meeting specific criteria. These were randomly allocated to one of three treatment groups. The control group (4th group) were self-selected, i.e. those patients who did not wish to have treatment or who could not attend for any reason. Patients received 3 hours a week of therapy for one year if possible. They were allocated to language orientation therapy, or to group stimulation therapy by speech therapists, or to group stimulation by other workers, e.g. nurses. The groups were stratified into type and severity of aphasia. The results showed that there was no significant difference between the treatment groups, however the comparison of all the treated subjects, i.e. the treatment types combined versus the untreated aphasic subjects, revealed a difference in that treatment was a significant factor in the amount of recovery. This is compounded by the fact that the control group were self selected and thus, may have been more ill, may have been less motivated, or may have had other difficulties. However, the control group had higher entry level scores on the assessments than the treated group, though they were comparable on aspects such as age, educational level, socio-economic status and aetiology. This study did not achieve the expected recruitment rate and had small numbers in each of the treatment groups. This had the result of increasing the true difference between groups necessary to show statistical significance. In this study when each treatment type was compared with each other type, no difference between them reached significance. A larger sample size might have determined whether there was a treatment of choice.

In the study above, the greatest language gains in both treated and untreated aphasic persons were made in the first few months, coinciding with the spontaneous recovery period. No significant differences between groups were evident and the slopes of the recovery curves were similar. In the second phase, the difference favoured the treated group, therefore the positive benefits of treatment were most apparent after the first 3 months. This time course of improvement was similar to that reported by Wertz *et al* (1981). Although no significant advantage for treatment was found in the first 3 months, the question of whether treatment in this period primes aphasic patients, so that they can take advantage of treatment later on, remains unknown.

In contrast to the many reports that claim language therapy for aphasics to be effective, only a few group studies have been published in which it explicitly states that aphasia therapy is not effective (Lincoln *et al.*, 1984; Richters *et al.*, 1976; Sarno *et al.*, 1970). The most convincing evidence in this respect has been presented by Lincoln *et al.* (1984) who randomly allocated 191 aphasic stroke patients to either speech therapy, receiving therapy twice a week for 24 weeks, or no-treatment control group. Although both groups showed some improvement on the Porch Index Communicative Ability (PICA) and the FCP, both standard aphasia tests, there were no significant differences in language recovery between the 104 patients allocated to the treatment group and the 87 patients of the control group. As the groups did not differ significantly on most variables that are believed to influence recovery (i.e. aetiology, time post-onset, type and severity of aphasia, age, and sex), these results suggest that individual speech and language therapy of the general stimulation type and of this intensity, does not improve language abilities more than is achieved by spontaneous recovery.

Understandably, this study stimulated a great deal of correspondence which claimed, among other things, that the subject selection criteria were inadequate, that too little treatment was provided to most patients and that the treatment methods themselves were insufficiently described (*Lancet*, 23 June 1984; Wertz *et al.*, 1986).

Although some of these criticisms seem justified, the design of the Lincoln study and in particular the random allocation of a large number of patients to treatment and no-treatment groups compares favourably with the ones used in most other studies in which significant therapy effects were reported.

Random control trials have come under criticism during the past few years (Howard, 1986; Pring, 1989). There is no doubt they pose difficulties to aphasiology. Prins, Schoonen and Vermeulen (1989) suggest that lack of attention to the internal validity and statistical power in the research design probably cause the conflicting conclusions in efficacy studies over the past three decades. Thought-provokingly, Fitz-Gibbon (1986) ponders whether RCTs would have been attacked so roundly if the results of these had been more positive. She argues that RCTs are the most appropriate methodology for testing hypotheses, but suggests a greater reliance on estimating Effect Sizes rather than statistical significance. Meta-analysis is a technique of research synthesis which does this. Whurr, Lorch and Nye (1992) synthesized the research findings of all the major group RCTs (45 studies) in aphasia to pool effect size and consider all variables that might affect outcome. The authors conclude that the verdict on the efficacy of treatment must remain open.

Late recovery studies

There are diverse views concerning the process of recovery in aphasia and the effects of speech and language therapy, ranging from confidence in the effectiveness of speech rehabilitation to the belief that language recovery is a function of physiological restitution (Lenneberg, 1967).

> 'The adult patient does not re-learn language. Neither training nor conditioning are guarantees for the restoration of language . . . There are reasons to believe that this is due to physiological restoration of function rather than the learning process.'

Shewan and Kertesz (1984) suggest that the efficacy question can be addressed without employing a no-treatment control group by using patients who are stable and beyond the period of spontaneous recovery, in order to investigate the ability to 'relearn'. Thus, gains in language function for patients after a period of language treatment could be attributed to the treatment provided. Dabul and Hanson (1975), reported significant language gains in the overall PICA scores of an aphasic patient group who had a mean post-onset duration of 14 months at treatment initiation. However the gains were significantly greater for a group who initiated treatment early, i.e at 1 month post onset. The authors do not state whether the groups were comparable at entry, although examination of the included data revealed no major discrepancies.

Broida (1977) also reported language gains in a group of aphasic patients initiating treatment at least 1 year post onset. Whether the improvement was statistically significant is not indicated.

A study, using a mixed group of aphasic patients, examined the effects of individual versus group treatment on recovery. Wertz *et al.* (1978, 1981) reported that both modes of therapy resulted in significant language gains during the year of treatment and significant gains were seen during the 26–48 week post-onset cohort, which is stated to be after the expected period of maximum spontaneous recovery. The groups were similar and where advantages did occur, they were in favour of those receiving individual treatment. Marked improvement, defined as a gain of 21 percentile points or more on the overall PICA scores, occurred in 83% of the patients treated individually as compared with 43% of the group treatment patients.

Again late recovery was reported by Aten, Caligiuri and Holland (1982), who evaluated the effectiveness of functional communication training with seven patients who had non-fluent agrammatic aphasia and had retained functional comprehension. These patients had had previous speech and language therapy and an average post-onset time of 97.9 months. The functional therapy is detailed and replicable but, in the current context of thinking on functional communication, appears somewhat dated. The test results on the PICA showed no significant change but a functional assessment (Communicative Abilities in Daily Living) revealed significant improvement in post-treatment performance, which was maintained at a 6 week follow-up.

Group studies comparing different modes of therapy delivery

Whether aphasic patients benefit from treatment may be disputed, but there appears to be general agreement that assessment, attention and support are appropriate (Benson, 1979; Darley, 1982). However, all persons who suffer aphasia do not receive even this. For some, no funds are available to support treatment (Collins, 1986). Other aphasic persons live too far from treatment centres to participate in treatment and frequently clinical case loads are too full to provide services for all aphasic patients who need them (Schuell *et al.*, 1964).

To combat funding, travel and personnel problems, the use of persons other than speech and language therapists to provide aphasia treatment has been examined (David *et al.*, 1982; Eaton-Griffith and Miller, 1980; Meikle *et al.*, 1979). This has also given a different method of forming a 'control' group.

Meikle *et al.* (1979) compared the progress of 16 aphasic patients, who received conventional treatment from speech therapists, with 15 patients treated by teams of volunteers. Patients not completing the treatment were excluded from results analysis. Comparisons of PICA scores revealed no significant difference in improvement between groups. However, several methodological limitations of the study, e.g. sample size and statistical validity confounded the results (Pring, 1989).

David, Enderby and Bainton (1982) also compared the progress of aphasic patients, treated by speech and language therapists, with patients treated by untrained volunteers. Of the 155 patients who entered, 96 received 30 hours of treatment over a span of 15–20 weeks. Progress was evaluated with two pre-treatment assessments, a week apart, four within treatment ratings at 2,4,8 and 12 weeks during treatment, and a post-test immediately after treatment. Results indicated that both groups improved but that there were no significant differences between groups on any evaluation. There was some indication that therapists had a better influence on outcome of more severely aphasic patients than had volunteers.

As in the Meikle study, methodological problems have been noted (Huber *et al.*, 1983; Pring, 1989). Wade (1983) argued that despite these studies using volunteers with aphasic patients, this did not support replacement of speech therapists by volunteers.

The *Lancet* editorial (1977) suggested that establishing the value of aphasia therapy is virtually impossible and outlined three complications when designing treatment studies. The first is that it is difficult to define a 'no-treatment group'. Many studies (Basso *et al.*, 1979; Hagen, 1973; Vignolo, 1964) have employed a 'self-selective no-treatment group' to avoid ethical problems but these produce difficulties by introducing unknown confounding aspects. Second, it is difficult to control biographical or medical variables that may influence response to treatment. Age, intelligence, education, aetiology, type of aphasia, time since onset, and environmental differences, cause difficulties. Finally, spontaneous recovery and improvement in language during the early period post onset, complicates controlled treatment trials.

The Veterans Administration (Wertz *et al.*, 1981) study attempts to 'respond to the *Lancet* editorial which suggests that there should be small, well-defined, groups comparing one mode of treatment with another and gradually building towards a hard-core of firm facts.' This study recruited 67 patients out of a possible aphasic population of 1071 who were screened. They were all male and randomly allocated to one of two treatment groups, receiving either individual treatment or group treatment. They had 8 hours of therapy each week which began 4 weeks post onset and continued for 48 weeks post onset. There was a high drop-out rate in both groups. Both groups made significant improvements in language abilities. Individual treatment resulted in significantly better overall performance on the PICA but no significant differences were observed between groups on the other language measures. Significant improvement in both groups, beyond 26 weeks post onset, indicated both individual and group treatment was an 'efficacious method of managing aphasic patients'.

One of the most carefully designed random controlled studies evaluating the efficacy of speech and language therapy for aphasia was again conducted, in the USA, by collaborating Veterans Administration Hospitals. This study by Marshall *et al.* (1989) selected 121 patients who fitted into very specific criteria from a possible 1800 referrals. These patients were randomly allocated to one of three groups: conventional treatment; treatment in the home, by a 'home volunteer', 'a trained spouse', 'other professional or volunteer'; and a group who had deferred therapy. The conventional treatment group made significantly more improvements than the deferred no-treatments group, but there was no significant difference between the conventionally treated group and the home treated group. The deferred treatment group 'caught up' when treated by speech pathologists later. 'We concluded from these results that speech pathology-treated patients made significantly more improvement than untreated patients' (Marshall *et al.*, 1989). The authors observed that volunteer-treated patients made more improvement than untreated patients on four of five outcome measures. More volunteer-treated patients made moderate to marked improvements on four of the five outcome measures than was displayed by patients who received no treatment. Fewer volunteer-treated patients became worse or showed no improvement on four of the five outcome measures when compared with the no-treatment group.

Combined group and single case studies

A new methodological approach was first used to evaluate aphasia therapy by Poeck, Huber and Willmes in 1989. This study compared, by means of psychometric single case analysis procedures, the outcome of aphasia in patients, receiving intensive language treatment (N = 68) with the amount of spontaneous improvement of a comparable group receiving no language treatment (N = 92), who had been studied previously in a nationwide study of the natural course of aphasia. Historical control groups may overcome the ethical difficulty of recruiting a control group but can give other methodological concerns such as independence and method of selecting the pair. The authors did not 'limit themselves to group comparisons'. By using a single case analysis they were able to assess the specific pattern of individual improvement.

The results indicated that, with intensive treatment, improvement went beyond that expected with spontaneous recovery in 78% of the patients treated up to 4 months post onset and in 46% of the patients treated 4–12 months post onset. 'It is possible these figures are too low because the correction procedures for accounting for spontaneous recovery were strict' (Poeck *et al.*, 1989). With intensive treatment, aphasia improved, 'even in the chronic stage, in 68% of the patients'. It appears that positive results were maintained at follow-up but inspection of the data shows that this follow-up included only a small number of 'chronic' patients. In this study, age, duration since onset, size and site of lesion and the impairment in intelligence, as assessed by standard tests, were not related to improvement. In the opinion of the authors, intensity and specificity of treatment appeared to be the crucial important factors. Specificity of treatment has not been considered in this way until this study.

A similar methodology was used by two authors in the previous study to compare two specific therapy approaches. PACE therapy (Davis and Wilcox, 1981) is pragmatically not linguistically orientated. Springer *et al.* (1991) compared the traditional PACE therapy with a modified PACE approach which incorporated training of lexical-semantic difficulties. Using a cross-over design convincing progress was demonstrated in three of the four subjects in general communication and naming.

Single case studies

The nature and type of speech and language deficits following stroke have attracted a great deal of research attention. Less attention has been paid to describing the therapists themselves and even less to analysing the actual process of therapy. Basso (1989) comments

> 'It is very difficult to know what aphasia therapy is . . . . What occurs under the heading of aphasia rehabilitation in one place may have nothing in common with what occurs in a different place except for the fact that a speech therapist and a patient interact with each other.'

The current neuropsychological emphasis espouses the interpretation of language deficits in terms of models of normal language processing. This has allowed hypotheses to be developed about the nature of language deficits, which have become acknowledged as prerequisites for detailed programmes of therapy, and allow greater clarity in describing goals of treatment. It is important that therapists know what to treat, in order that they may evaluate the response of the patient and modify therapy accordingly. However, 'knowing what is wrong does not, in any simple way, determine what to do about it' (Howard and Hatfield, 1987).

Single case analysis has been closely linked to evaluating this method of treatment and allows inspection of individual characteristics of aphasic behaviour and treatment.

> 'One of the important aspects of carrying out single case studies of the effectiveness of therapy, is that the therapy should be replicable so that if a treatment method proves successful with one patient then it may be repeated with another similarly impaired patient' (Byng, 1988).

Byng (1988) gave an account of therapy to remediate a specific sentence processing deficit in an individual patient. Nickels, Byng and Black (1991) undertook a replication of this therapy with a patient who had similar although not identical deficits to those of another patient, JG, described in the earlier study. The patient in this study was a monolingual English male, aged 65 years, and was 3 years post-stroke. The therapy was performed using tasks which retained the key theoretical motivating principles, but differed in detail due to individual differences between the patients. Sentence comprehension and production both improved as a result of therapy. The pattern of results observed give further insight into both the nature of the patient's deficit and the mechanism for therapy, the patient improving significantly on those tasks predicted but not on unrelated tasks.

Hillis (1989) used a similar approach to inspect the treatment of two aphasic patients who both made frequent semantic errors in verbal picture naming and errors in written naming. Different patterns of errors, across various language tasks provided evidence that the two patients' naming errors arose from different underlying deficits. The effectiveness of cueing hierarchies on improving each patient's written naming was demonstrated in single subject experiments using a multiple base line design. Although both patients exhibited acquisition and maintenance of written naming, only one showed generalization to verbal naming and to untrained stimuli. These different results are interpreted as a reflection of separate underlying deficits leading to the subject's naming errors. The authors suggest that determining the cognitive basis of an individual's naming difficulty may permit predictions concerning language behaviours that are likely to improve concurrently.

A similar detailed approach by Wambaugh and Thompson (1989) was taken to study four Brocas aphasic subjects using a multiple baseline design to evaluate the stimulus and response generalization effect of training WH-Interrogative Production (use of 'what', 'where' questions). Throughout treatment, response generalization to untrained questions and stimulus generalization to several non-training conditions were assessed. Results indicate that 'questions production treatment' facilitates the production of trained 'what, where' constructions. The level of the improved production varied slightly amongst the subjects. Whilst all the subject's responses, during treatment, exceeded those observed during base line there was variable response generalization to untrained items and little generalization to grammatically different constructions. The response generalization results reveal that treatment applied to 'what' interrogatives did not facilitate production of 'where' interrogatives and vice-versa. This limited generalization may be attributable to the therapy: '. . . where there are good psycholinguistic reasons for generalization . . . to take place, and when these are made explicit and incorporated within therapy, then generalization can take place'.

A study using multiple baseline design assessed the effects of a generalization training procedure on the ability of four subjects with chronic aphasia (29–195 months post onset) to make requests (Doyle *et al.*, 1989). Generalization and use of the behaviour was greater with the trainers than with unfamiliar volunteers. Nevertheless all the subjects' requests increased with all conversational participants to a level of that of a normal comparison group assessed under identical conditions.

Difficulty with repetition is viewed as a primary deficit in conduction aphasia. Consequently repetition is considered to be a target of treatment as opposed to an approach to treatment for this syndrome (Kohn *et al.*, 1990). CM, the patient in this study, started his programme 7 months post onset. After 2 months of 'repetition treatment', CM displayed significant improvement in his sentence repetition both in terms of number of content words that he produced correctly and the portion of sentences that he produced correctly. These improvements generalized to other speech contexts but the relevance to everyday communication was not detailed.

The importance of targeting therapy to the hypothesized underlying deficit in order to test the hypothesis as well as increasing the likelihood of benefit was postulated by Jones (1986) who described a therapeutic programme for a non-fluent patient who had not improved after 6 years of therapy, when his sentence construction impairments were reconsidered in the light of current theoretical hypotheses. Whilst this case description has weaknesses, the targeted therapy appears to achieve accessibility to the patients sentence mapping abilities. A more rigorous study examines this question in detail and appears to confirm Jones's finding.

Frequently in clinical practice a particular treatment approach for a particular aphasic disorder may be used indiscriminately despite the possibility of different underlying disorders. Nettleton and Lesser (1991), using repeated case study design with six aphasic patients, examined whether 'model appropriate therapy' was more effective than 'model inappropriate therapy'. Three of the four subjects receiving model appropriate therapy showed improvement after 8 weeks of therapy; the two subjects receiving 'model inappropriate therapy' did not improve.

The strength of single case and small group studies is in the detail of particular approaches to treatment. Sufficient information can be given in the papers so that the treatment approaches can be replicated and details of the subjects would help selection of the right patient for proven methods. The suggestion that specificity of treatment is a crucial factor appears to be supported by the few studies undertaken so far (Byng and Lesser, 1993).

Evaluation of other therapies for aphasia

Whilst counselling for aphasia should not be considered as a novel approach, the thought that it should be compared with traditional speech and language therapy, perhaps, is a new one as the component of counselling in traditional therapy may itself be quite large.

The study by Hartman, William and Landau (1987) randomly assigned 60 sequential aphasic patients to receiving either speech and language therapy or counselling. These authors concluded that conventional SLT therapy offered no more than the general support offered by counselling. However, Wertz (1988) criticized the study on the randomization technique, the lack of detail regarding treatment intensity and mixing aetiologies, and the interpretation of results which he felt indicated a significant improvement in the speech and language therapy group.

The wide range of speech therapy techniques is demonstrated by the following studies. The first by Whitney and Goldstein (1989) assessed the effects of treatment designed to teach mildly aphasic individuals to monitor dysfluencies, revisions, repetitions and audible pauses in their connected speech. Treatment effects were evaluated using a multiple base line design across three subjects. All subjects showed immediate and dramatic reductions in the frequency of these behaviours in the picture description task when self-monitoring was introduced. Two subjects simultaneously reduced un-targeted dysfluencies and all three generalized their improved speech to another task. Treatment effects were unrelated to the accuracy of self-monitoring. The improved speech was characterized by a slower speaking rate, but more efficient communication, as reflected by longer, uninterrupted utterances. Standardized test scores were unchanged but unfamiliar listeners found perceptible improvement between base line and post-treatment audio tapes.

Gardner *et al.* (1976) introduced a visual communication system which associated simple geometric forms and line drawings with particular meanings. Only 2 out of 15 patients could use the symbol system after it was taught spontaneously to convey immediate needs. Blissymbolics, Amerind and pictograms have also been taught and all have proved difficult to evaluate when considering the concept of extending communication beyond the immediate context. However, Bertoni, Stoffel and Weniger (1991) described a case study of a 58-year-old man, with severe aphasia following a stroke, who after 18 months of conventional therapy, had hardly improved his verbal expression and was introduced to therapy using pictograms. The case study describes how the patient developed his attempts so that he was able to express himself by drawing pictograms. These 'appeared to convey the intended message quite convincingly but often remain ambiguous with a considerable degree of intuition on the part of the listener'.

Many speech and language therapists state that one of their goals is to assist other carers to understand the patients' difficulties and to encourage strategies that facilitate communication. Two quasi experimental studies have reported evaluation in this area (Buckwalter *et al.*, 1988, 1989). The studies demonstrated the benefits of an individual communication enhancement programme, devised by the SLT, for elderly ward-based patients. The programmes were implemented by nurses for 10 minutes a day during the course of daily care, e.g. making the bed or dressing the resident. The studies acknowledge confounding factors that limit confidence in the findings but there is sufficient evidence to suggest that this approach should be considered further. Evaluating the value of programmes designed by SLTs but, in this instance, delivered by relatives was the objective of an investigation conducted by Lesser *et al.* (1986). The programme was based on a detailed approach developed by Salonen (1980) reflecting Luria's approach 'Reacquisition of language in aphasia depends on the reintegration of the linguistic systems and on the restoration of the interactions between language and other mental functions'. The regime involved 1 hour per week with the therapist and an average of 5 hours per week with the relative over a period of 3 months. Seven of the nine patients were reported on and showed marked improvement on the Western Aphasia Battery.

Speech and language therapy combined with pharmacological therapy

There have been various trials over the last 30 years to establish whether aphasia can be improved by drugs. Anti-depressants and muscle relaxants were amongst the first that were advocated although no significance trials were conducted at the time. A more recent study, in 1990, by Capon, Lehert and Opsomer investigated the use of Natfidro-Furyl in the treatment of sub-acute stroke. This study was a double blind random controlled study of 82 patients in the sub-acute phase of stroke. Patients were excluded who were likely to make a spontaneous recovery requiring discharge in 1 month, and also those who were likely to die. Those treated with Natfidro-Furyl showed a statistically significant improvement for walking and activities of daily living, as compared to the group treated by a placebo, but there was no difference for aphasic patients on expression or comprehension. However, the study does not mention the assessments that were used. Improvement was negatively influenced by age, and all scores except psychometric scores, showed improvement for the active drug treatment, compared with the placebo, even though some of these were not significant.

There have been several studies to investigate the effectiveness of Piracetam, which is a neurotropic agent, specifically with aphasia. In one study, reported by Poeck, Huber and Willmes in 1993, patients were randomly assigned to receive placebo or Piracetam. The groups were comparable at baseline. Significant difference was found in favour of the Piracetam group for the 'profile height' which is a weighting of the sum scores of the different sub-tests of the Aachen Aphasia Test. Whilst all the sub-tests improved more under Piracetam treatment than under the placebo, the specific differences for the sub-tests 'written language' and 'token test' reached, respectively, significance and trend level. In general, patients improved twice as much under Piracetam as under placebo whilst receiving the same amount of intensive speech and language therapy.

Conclusion

A detailed investigation into the factors affecting the prognosis of aphasia analysed retrospective base line information of 110 sequentially referred patients who met certain criteria, who were selected from a cohort of a possible 500 (Marshall *et al.*, 1982). Base line severity was accounted for and the findings suggested that those who do well are younger, in better health and start therapy earlier. Those who do not do so well tend to be older, initially more severe, have had thrombo-embolic strokes, and have poorer comprehension. The most predictive characteristics of treatment responsiveness were: treatment intensity, time of treatment after onset, and age. The authors warn that this data should not be construed to indicate that the more treatment patients receive, the more recovery they will make. It is likely that patients who are more responsive are offered more treatment because they are able to participate in the treatment process itself.

However, a relationship between the amount of treatment and outcome of intervention *is* suggested in some reports. Wertz *et al.* (1986) who provided programmes for 8 hours per week for up to 44 weeks, noted that those treated for longer progressed more. Where treatment has been provided at a rate of at least three sessions per week, and has continued for not less than 5 months, a positive outcome has been reported (Basso *et al.*, 1979; Shewan and Kertesz, 1984). Basso and her co-workers (1979) have recommended at least 6 months of therapy with a minimum of three sessions weekly.

> 'Durations of therapy have varied from four weeks to one year. Intensity has been found to be equally variable with ranges from three sessions of probably one hour each per week to five hours per day and 25 hours per week.'

It is regrettable, for the many thousands of aphasia sufferers, that therapy has often been reduced to negligible amounts. The fact that intervention can be helpful may no longer be in question but the amount of treatment necessary for maximum benefit to be derived needs to be established. Two sessions of two hours per week, considered typical of clinical practice, has been a popular therapy regime in research, but Lincoln *et al.* (1984) and Prins, Schoonen and Vermeulen (1989) found that 5 months of this treatment frequency was not advantageous when treated and untreated groups were compared.

Mackenzie (1991) concluded that clinicians may not consider intensive therapy as an option, despite its apparent efficacy, due to resource limitations. However, it seems that when taking into account factors such as interest, willingness, and general health, the number of subjects for whom intensive treatment is feasible is not great (Leigh-Smith *et al.* 1987). There needs to be a radical reorganization of current provision if therapy is to be effective with chronic aphasia and if we are to base our service on the knowledge currently available (David and Enderby, 1990).

Many research studies have concentrated primarily on whether treatment achieves positive gains in language function, but the nature, duration and intensity of this treatment have received comparatively little attention (Shewan and Kertesz, 1984). It is unfortunate that so many reports have contained so little information on treatment methods used and other studies have not attempted to control it.

> 'The exact content of the therapy session was highly variable dependent on the patient and treatment centre and the speech therapist involved' (Prins *et al.*, 1978).

Four recent group studies and all but one single case study, report favourable effects of language treatment. Of the group studies, three were conducted in single clinical institutions with restricted selection of patients and homogenous methods of treatment (Basso *et al.*, 1979; Shewan and Kertesz, 1984; Wertz *et al.*, 1981). The most recent study (Wertz *et al.*, 1986) was conducted in five VA hospitals with high frequency treatment and rigid entry criteria. In contrast there have been negative reports from earlier multi-centre studies concluding that general non-specific low intensity treatment, directly provided by professionals, whilst effective is not superior to volunteer treatment (David *et al.*, 1982; Meikle *et al.*, 1979). Furthermore, Hartman, William and Landau (1987), reported professional counselling to be as efficient as direct language treatment. One study claims that language treatment has no effect at all (Lincoln *et al.*, 1984).

Wertz (1987) suggests that whether aphasia therapy is efficacious is no longer the important question! The present issue that requires investigation is related to the selection of patients who will benefit, at what time, with which specific therapy and what amount. In a review of the literature he suggests that the aphasic who will benefit is likely to have a single, left hemisphere thromboembolic infarct with moderate aphasia of 3 months or less onset who can receive 3 hours treatment a week for at least 5 months.

All workers in this field are faced with the question as to what constitutes good recovery, and whilst there are many standardized tests of language function, these may not inform us regarding the efficiency, effectiveness, naturalness of a person's communication and his or her ability to cope with life.

Sarno, Sarno and Levita (1971) compared a functional communication quotient (FCQ) with a formal test (NCCEA). The comparison revealed that improvement, on parts of the objective test (NCCEA) has not always accompanied useful improvements as measured by the functional test. Despite this insight, published more than 20 years ago, there are still few acceptable ways of analysing communication ability in its broader sense. Whilst conversational analysis may have something to offer in the future we have, as a profession, few measures to assess the ultimate goal, i.e. general communication. The statement that 'Arguably any improvement on a series of formal language tests is quite meaningless as long as this improvement does not express itself in the communicative interactions of daily living' (Prins et al., 1978) remains a challenge today.

Furthermore, the role of the speech and language therapist tends to be substantially broader than that which is immediately apparent. For example, the SLT not only aims to remediate speech and language but also has a role in facilitating autonomy of the patient, supporting and informing the patient and relatives, improving non-verbal communication, etc, and these aspects have not been clearly described or evaluated (Brumfitt, 1985; Holland and Beeson, 1993). Most aphasia studies have used standardized aphasia tests to measure outcome, yet these tests may be measuring little or nothing that has been targeted in therapy. Thus, changes in these measures would not be expected, whilst changes in other measures may have been expected (Byng et al., 1989), and therefore the efficacy of aphasia rehabilitation as a whole still requires further attention.

A step in this direction, which may in the future be viewed as the beginning of a trend into psychosocial qualitative research in this field, was undertaken by Ireland, herself aphasic and Wootton (Ireland and Balck, 1992; Ireland and Wootton, 1993). The object was to set up counselling services for aphasics and examine how this helped. The study resulted in the recommendation that counselling services should be available to aphasics, as it was generally viewed as valuable and desirable. It may appear strange that describing, recording and quantifying events that contribute to therapy have attracted so little attention. This could be linked to the medical perspective of research in aphasia – usually treatments in medicine require little unpacking; drugs and procedures are frequently not so easily influenced by personal perspective or interpretation. Whilst methods of describing and recording therapy were suggested by Brookshire, Nicholas and Kreuger in 1978, the relevance to efficacy research has only recently been raised.

'A whole new set of questions need to be asked about therapy to determine how it works and to clarify what we are trying to do through therapy' (Byng, 1993).

References

Aten J, Caligiuri MP and Holland A (1982). The efficacy of functional communication therapy for chronic aphasic patients. Journal of Speech and Hearing Disorders 47: 93–96.

Basso A, Capitani E, and Vignolo LA (1979). Influence of rehabilitation in language skills in aphasic patients: A controlled study. Archives of Neurology 36: 190–196.

Basso A (1989). Spontaneous recovery in language rehabilitation. In: Seron X, Deloche G (Eds) Cognitive Approaches in Neuropsychological Rehabilitation. Hillsdale, NY: Lawrence Erlbaum.

Beaton A, Davidoff J and Erstfeld V (1991). An opticaphasis and visual agnosia (translation and commentary on Freund 1889). Cognitive Neuropsychology 8: 21–39.

Benson DF (1979). Aphasic rehabilitation. Archives of Neurology 36: 187–189.

Bertoni B, Stoffel AM and Weniger D (1991) Communicating with pictographs: A graphic approach to the improvement of communicative interactions. Aphasiology. 5(4, 5): 341–353.

Broida H (1977). Language therapy effects in long term aphasia. Archives of Physical Medicine and Rehabilitation 58: 248–253.

Brookshire R, Nicholas L and Kreuger K (1978). Sampling of speech pathology treatment activities. An evaluation of momentary and interval sampling procedures. Journal of Speech and Hearing Research 21: 652–667.

Brumfitt S (1985). Another side to therapy. CST Bulletin No 397.

Buckwalter KC, Cusack D, Sidles E, Wadle K and Beaver M (1988). The behavioral consequences of a communication intervention on institutionalised residents with aphasia and dysarthria. Archives of Psychiatric Nursing 11(5): 289–295.

Buckwalter KC, Cusack D, Sidles E, Wadle K and Beaver M (1989). Increasing communication ability in aphasic/dysarthric patients. Western Journal of Nursing Research 11(6): 736–747.

Butfield E and Zangwill OL (1946). Re-education in aphasia: Review of 70 cases. Journal of Neurology, Neurosurgery and Psychiatry 9: 75–79.

Byng S (1988). Sentence processing deficits: theory and therapy. Cognitive Neuropsychology 5(6): 629–676.

Byng S (1993). Hypotheses testing and aphasia therapy. In: Holland A and Forbes M (Eds) Aphasia Treatment: World Perspectives, 124. London: Chapman & Hall.

Byng S, Kay J, Edmundson B and Scott T (1989). Aphasia tests reconsidered. Aphasiolgy. 4(1): 67–91.

Byng S and Lesser R (1993). A review of therapy at the level of the sentence in aphasia. In: Paradis M (Ed.) Foundation of Aphasia Rehabilitation, IALP. Oxford: Pergamon Press.

Capon A, Lehert P, and Opsomer L (1990). Natfidro-furyl in the treatment of subacute stroke. Journal of Cardiovascular Pharmacology 16 (suppl 3): S62–S66. .

Collins M (1986). Diagnosis and Treatment of Global Aphasia. London: Taylor & Francis.

Dabul B and Hanson WR (1975). The amount of language improvement in adult aphasics related to early and late treatment. Paper presented at the Annual Convention of the American Speech and Hearing Association. Washington DC. November.(As quoted in Shewan and Kertesz.)

Darley F (1982). Aphasia. Philadelphia: WB Saunders.

David R and Enderby P (1990). Speech therapy – operating a rationed service. Clinical Rehabilitation 4(3): 245–253.

David RM, Enderby P and Bainton D (1982). Progress report on an evaluation of speech therapy for aphasia. British Journal of Disorders of Communication 14(2): 85–88.

Davis G and Wilcox M (1981). Incorporating parameters of natural conversation in aphasia treatment. In: Chapey R (Ed) Language Intervention Strategies in Adult Aphasia. Baltimore, MD: Williams and Wilkins.

Davis GA and Wilcox MJ (1985). Adult Aphasia Rehabilitation. San Diego, CA: College Hill Press.

Doyle P, Goldstein H, Bourgeois M and Nakles K (1989). Facilitating generalised requesting behaviour in Broca's aphasia: An experimental analysis of a generalisation training procedure. Journal of Applied Behaviour Analysis 22(2): 157–170.

Eaton-Griffith VE and Miller C (1980). Volunteer stroke scheme for dysphasic patients with stroke. British Medical Journal 281: 1605–1607.

Enderby P and Davies P (1989). Communication disorders: Planning a service to meet the needs. British Journal of Disorders of Communication 24: 301–331.

Fitz-Gibbon CT (1986). In defence of randomised controlled trials, with suggestions about the possible use of meta-analysis. British Journal of Disorders of Communication 21: 117–124.

Gardner H, Zurif E, Berry T and Baker E (1976). Visual communication in aphasia. Neuropsychologia 14: 275–292.

Godfrey CM and Douglass E (1959). The recovery process in aphasia. Canadian Medical Association Journal 80: 618–624.

Hagen C (1973). Communication abilities in hemiplegia: Effect of speech therapy. Archives of Physical Medicine and Rehabilitation 54: 454 -463.

Hartman J, William M and Landau M (1987). Comparison of formal language therapy with supportive counselling for aphasia due to acute vascular accident. Archives of Neurology 44: 646–649.

Hillis AE. (1989). Efficacy and generalization of treatment for aphasic naming errors. Archives of Physical Medicine Rehabilitation 70: 632–636.

Holland AL and Beeson PM (1993). Finding a new sense of self: what the clinician can do to help. Aphasiology 7(6): 581–583.

Howard D (1986). Beyond randomised controlled trials: The case for effective case studies of the effect of treatment in aphasia. British Journal of Disorder of Communication 21: 89–102.

Howard D and Hatfield FM (1987). Aphasia Therapy: Historical and Contemporary Issues. London: Lawrence Earlbaum.

Huber W, Poeck K, Wenigar D and Willmes K (1983). Der Aachener Aphasietest. Göttingen: Verlag fr psycholigie.

Ireland C and Black M (1992). Living with aphasia: The insight story. Working Papers in Linguistics 4. London: University College.

Ireland C and Wootton G (1993). Action for Dysphasic Adults Counselling Project 'Time to Talk'. DOH Report.

Jones E (1986). Building the foundations for sentence production in a non-fluent aphasic. British Journal of Disorders of Communication 21: 63–82.

Keenan J and Brassell E (1973). A study of factors related to prognosis for individual aphasic patients. Journal of Speech and Hearing Disorders 39: 257–269.

Kohn S, Smith K and Arsenault J (1990). The remediation of conduction aphasia via sentence repetition: a case study. British Journal of Disorders of Communication 25: 45–60.

Lancet (1977). Progress in aphasia. Editorial. 2: 24.

Lancet (1984). Letter page. Speech therapy for aphasic stroke patients. 23 June, 1413–1414.

La Pointe L L (1977). Base-10 Programmed-Stimulation: Task specification scoring and plotting performance in aphasia therapy. Journal of Speech and Hearing Disorders 42: 90–105.

Leigh-Smith J, Denis R, Enderby P, Wade D and Langton Hewer R (1987). Selection of aphasic stroke patients for intensive speech therapy. Journal of Neurology, Neurosurgery and Psychiatry 50: 1488–1492.

Lenneberg EH (1967). The Biological Foundations of Language. New York: Wiley.

Lesser R, Bryan K, Anderson J and Hilton R (1986). Involving relatives in aphasia therapy: An application of language enrichment therapy. International Journal of Rehabilitation Research 9(3): 259–267.

Lincoln NB, Mulley GP, Jones AC, McGuirk E, Lendrem W and Mitchell J (1984). Effectiveness of speech therapy for aphasic stroke patients: a randomised control trial. Lancet 1: 1197–1200.

Lyon JG (1992). Communication use and participation in life for adults with aphasia in natural settings: The scope of the problem. American Journal of Speech and Language Pathology 1: 7–15.

Mackenzie C (1991). An aphasia group intensive efficacy study. British Journal of Disorders of Communication 26: 275–291.

Marks M, Taylor M and Rusk H (1957). Rehabilitation of the aphasic patient: A survey of three years experience in a rehabilitation setting. Archives of Physical Medicine and Rehabilitation 38: 219–226.

Marshall RC, Tompkins CA and Phillips D (1982). Improvement in treated aphasia: An examination of selected prognostic factors. Folia Phoniatrica 34(6): 305–315.

Marshall RC, Wertz RT, Weiss DG, Aten JL, Brookshire RH, Garcia-Bunuel L, Holland A, Kurtzke J, La Pointe L, Milinti F, Brannegan R, Greenbaum H, Vogel D, Carter J, Barnes N and Goodman R (1989). Home treatment for aphasic patients by trained non-professionals. Journal of Speech and Hearing Disorders 54: 462–470.

Meikle M, Wechsler E, Tupper A, Benenson M, Butler J, Mulhall D and Stern G (1979). Comparative trial of volunteer and professional treatment of aphasia after stroke. British Medical Journal 2: 87–89.

Nettleton J and Lesser R (1991). Therapy for naming difficulties in aphasia: Application of a cognitive neuropsychological model. Journal of Neurolinguistics 6(2): 139–157.

Nickels L, Byng S and Black M (1991). Sentence processing deficits: a replication of therapy. British Journal of Disorders of Communication 26: 175–199.

Poeck K, Huber W and Willmes K (1989). Outcome of intensive language treatment in aphasia. Journal of Speech and Hearing Disorders 54: 471–479.

Poeck K, Huber W and Willmes K (1993). Piracetam as an add-on treatment to intensive speech therapy for aphasia. Abstract: 2nd International Conference on Stroke. Geneva, May.

Pring TR (1989). Evaluating the effects of speech therapy for aphasics and volunteers: Developing the single case methodology. British Journal of Disorders of Communication 21: 103–115.

Prins RS, Schoonen R and Vermeulen J (1989). Efficacy of two different types of speech therapy for aphasic stroke patients. Applied Psycholinguistics 10(1): 85–123.

Prins RS, Snow CE and Wagenaar E (1978). Recovery from aphasia: Spontaneous speech versus language comprehension. Brain and Language 6: 192–211.

Richters H, Wagenaar E, Houwen I and Spaans L (1976). Het herstelverloop van afasie. Een psycholinguistich onderzoek uitegevoerd in opdracht van de stichting Afasie. Nederland 1971–1975 Amsterdam:S.A.N.

Salonen L (1980). The language enriched individual therapy programme for aphasic adults. In: Taylor-Sarno M, Hook O (Eds) Aphasia Assessment and Treatment. Stockholm: Almqvist and Wiksall.

Sarno MT, Silverman M and Sands E (1970). Speech therapy and language recovery in severe aphasia. Journal of Speech and Hearing Research 13: 607–623.

Sarno JE, Sarno MT and Levita E (1971). Evaluating language improvement after completed stroke. Archives of Physical Medicine and Rehabilitation 52: 73–78.

Schuell H, Jenkins JJ and Jiminez-Pabon E (1964). Aphasia in Adults: diagnosis, prognosis and treatment. New York: Harper and Row.

Shewan CM and Kertesz A (1984). Effects of speech and language treatment on recovery from aphasia. Brain and Language 23: 272–299.

Springer L, Glindemann R, Huber W and Willmes K (1991). How efficacious is PACE-therapy when 'language systematic training' is incorporated? Aphasiology 5(4,5): 391–399.

Vignolo LA (1964). Evaluation of aphasia and language rehabilitation: A retrospective exploratory study. Cortex 1: 344–367.

Wade DT (1983). Can aphasic patients with stroke do without a speech therapist? British Medical Journal 286: 50.

Wambaugh J and Thompson C (1989). Training and generalisation of agrammatic aphasic adults. WH-Interrogative Productions. Journal of Speech and Hearing Disorders 54: 509–525.

Wertz RT (1987). Language treatment for aphasia is efficacious, but for whom? Topics of Language Disorders 8(1): 1–10.

Wertz RT (1988). A letter to the editor. Archives of Neurology 45: 372.

Wertz RT, Collins MJ, Weiss D, Kurtzke JF, Frieden T, Brookshire RH, Pierce J, Holtzapple P, Hubbard DJ. Porch BE, West JA, Davis L, Matovitch V, Morley GK and Resurrecion E (1978). Preliminary report on a comparison of individual and group treatment. Paper Presented at the Annual Meeting of the American Association for the Advancement of Science, Washington DC. (As reported in Shewan and Kertesz.)

Wertz RT, Collins MJ, Weiss D, Kurtzke JF, Frieden T, Brookshire RH, Pierce J, Holtzapple P, Hubbard DJ. Porch BE, West JA, Davis L, Matovitch V, Morley GK and Resurrecion E (1981). Veterans administration cooperation study on aphasia: A comparison of individual and group treatment. Journal of Speech and Hearing Research 24: 580–594.

Wertz RT, Weiss DG, Aten J, Brookshire RH, Garcia-Bunuel L, Holland A, Kurtzke JF, La Pointe L, Milianti F, Branegan R, Greenbaum H, Marshall R, Vogel D, Carter J, Barnes N and Goodman R (1986). Comparison of clinic, home, and deferred language treatment for aphasia: Veterans Administration Cooperation Study. Archives of Neurology 43: 653–658.

Whitney J and Goldstein H (1989). Using self-monitoring to reduce disfluency in speakers with mild aphasia. Journal of Speech and Hearing Disorders 54: 576–586.

Whurr R, Lorch MP and Nye C (1992). A meta-analysis of studies carried out between 1946 and 1988 concerned with the efficacy of speech and language therapy treatment for aphasic patients. European Journal of Disorders of Communication 27(1): 1–17.

Chapter 3
Children with Speech and Language Disorders

Introduction

Children are referred to Speech and Language Therapists for a number of reasons. They may be delayed in starting to speak or in progressing in the development of expressive or receptive language, or have delayed or deviant articulation, phonology, fluency or voice (Ingram 1972). Ingram cautions readers that before estimates of the prevalence of disorders of speech in childhood are accepted, the criteria of what constitutes a speech defect and the methods of selection, should be reviewed with care.

The normal acquisition of speech and language shows considerable variation and it is not always easy to distinguish between a child at the lower range of normality and one who is deviating from the usual pattern of speech and language development.

Prevalence

The pioneering work of Morley (1972), which was cited and used in the Quirk report (1972), found that 14% of 5-year-old children had serious articulatory defects, of which 4% were unintelligible to their teachers. The National Child Development Study (Butler *et al.*, 1973; Peckham, 1973), found that between 10% and 13% of 7-year-old children had some degree of speech impairment. These were more often males and children from manual backgrounds. Teachers in this study reported 10.7% of the children to be difficult to understand because of poor speech. An average of these estimates suggests that 12.1% of early school-age children have speech or language problems which may be a consequence of pathology or delay.

A more recent survey conducted by British Telecom for Speakwatch (1994), a public awareness campaign, elicited that 20% of mothers were concerned about the speech and language development of their pre-school children. Enderby and Davies (1989) deduced that, approximately

968 children per 100 000 population between the ages of 3 and 9 years have a speech or language problem that warrants the attention of a speech therapist.

Issues Affecting Efficacy Studies

In the 1930s and 1940s, children who had difficulty with developing speech and language were thought to have a common problem (Heltman, 1936). The primary disorder was labelled dyslalia,which was thought to be related to an inability for the ear to 'discriminate between different sounds'. Research over the last 20 years has offered many different theories for the various types of speech and language delays and disorders. Psycholinguistics, sociolinguistics, neurolinguistics, psychology and educational research have all contributed much to our understanding. However, there remain many theoretical conflicts, which leads to difficulties regarding classification of children with these problems and hypotheses for treatment.

Some themes seem to have run through the history of therapy. It was recognized very early on, and has continued to be emphasized, that language is acquired in a social context through a process made possible by the communication that occurs during social interaction. The importance of the social context in therapy also has been emphasized (Snow *et al.*, 1984).

Whilst each chapter in this volume addresses difficulties of efficacy research related to speech and language therapy, there is no other client group in this review that demonstrates so many challenges to the researcher. The heterogeneity of the client group, the range of presenting deficits, and the inadequate information on the natural history of speech and language development is compounded by a debate about discrimination between delayed and deviant speech and language, and thus presents a daunting prospect. This is further complicated by the lack of agreement relating to terminology, inadequately described therapy approaches and problems related to assessment.

It is beyond the scope of this paper to go into detail regarding the current discourse about speech and language development and the nature of the various disorders. However, there are some issues that should be highlighted as they impinge heavily on the type of therapy available and its evaluation.

Heterogeneity/normal development

There is unresolved debate regarding description of the cohort of children who would be defined as having speech and language impairment/specific language impairment, or phonological or pragmatic disorders. Whilst there has been a rapid increase in the knowledge base regarding the normal development of speech and language, which underpins different theoretical and philosophical principles about the nature of language and its interrelationship, these are still embryonic and have not fully informed the development of therapy procedures.

Determining whether a child has a general developmental delay or learning disability, or a specific difficulty in learning skills related to communication, is more problematic than first appears. Judith Johnson (1985) reminds us that the language–mind relationship does not work in one direction only and that, during the acquisition period, children use their available language skills to represent absent objects and events. One can speculate, therefore, that children who are language impaired at a certain stage find it increasingly difficult to follow the normal language maturation process. Despite this, she argues that in these children, language acquisition, although late and slow, is not 'off course' and does not violate any of the tenets of child language theory: 'it is a rule formulated process and learned in the course of communication events'. Her work suggests a similar relationship between thought and language, use of language for a variety of social purposes, and the normal sequence in rule formation to generate novel utterances, to reveal knowledge of abstract linguistic patterns. Johnson feels that the main problem with this particular group of children is that they are remarkably slow in the discovery of language patterns and a key symptom of the language disorder is a development gap between language knowledge and achievement in other areas of learning, for example conceptual, social, motor and perceptual.

Terminology

There is a lack of consensus and clarity relating to terminology. Authors do not describe children in similar ways and it is possible, if not likely, that different features predominate in different studies. Those referred to by Johnson (1967) may very well be of a specific type that show the maturational lag and difficulty in focusing on and learning language as discussed previously. These seem to be essentially a different group from those who have other associated problems described by other authors. In an attempt to define groups more clearly to overcome some of these difficulties Stark and Tallal (1981) defined some exclusion criteria for specific language impairment. These criteria ensure that the children's language problem is of primary nature rather than secondary and they are defined as 'not having a hearing loss, significant emotional or behavioral problems, below average intelligence, neurological problems or oral defect'. Although these criteria are widely used, some research studies have not adhered to them, notably the work of Bishop and colleagues (see Adams and Bishop, 1989; Bishop and Adams, 1989; Bishop and Adams, 1992; Bishop and Edmundson, 1987). These authors use the term 'specific language impairment' (SLI) to refer to children who present primary language disorders rather than language problems secondary to some known aetiology, but do not exclude children with histories of significant recurrent otitis media or neurological disease.

Some of the reasons for lack of precision in criteria is that many children have more than one difficulty. For example, children with marked phonological, along with syntactic or semantic, deficits are not currently labelled 'SLI' consistent with the practices of Stark and Tallal (1981). However, much research focusing on SLI, since that time, still fails to characterize the receptive skills of subjects precisely and does not use severity and specificity as bases for exclusion and inclusion.

A survey by Nye and Weems (1991) of 103 research studies of language-disordered children attempted to determine the nature and characteristics of the identification criteria represented. Five categories of language disorder identification criteria were found. These were:

Discrepancy: 14% of the studies reported a discrepancy required for subject participation, i.e. a discrepancy of language development against mental age. Some of these used a 6 month discrepancy, some used a 1 year discrepancy, others used standard deviations.

Exclusion: an exclusionary statement was reported in 40% of the studies representing a total of 15 different exclusion classifications. For example, hearing impairment, mental retardation, neurological handicap, visual handicap.

Intelligence: 17 studies identified subjects on the basis of intelligence scores.

Subject setting: an analysis of the setting from which subjects were recruited revealed five divisions: school settings, clinical settings, home settings, university settings, and various settings.

Focus of study: the majority of the studies surveyed dealt with various dimensions of language across five areas (65%). Most research attention was directed towards the area of *semantics*, with a total of 45 studies reporting data in this area. The second most frequent studied area was *syntax* (35 studies), followed by *phonology* (19 studies), *pragmatics* (13 studies) and *psycholinguistics* (13 studies).

In Nye and Weem's review, over 50 different language instruments were used in the studies surveyed. The authors conclude that the published research on child language disorders suggests a diverse perspective on language disorders that detracts from the narrowing of the focus of language disorders and results in a heterogenous sample of children receiving the same label. Thus the term, 'language disorders', applies to a widely varying population.

Natural history of speech and language impairments

Speech and language skills are known to develop throughout life and it is likely that speech and language disorders, without intervention, would change in their nature and severity. However, there is little information in the literature regarding the natural history of the disorders that would set into context the efforts of therapeutic programmes. Such studies that have been carried out do not specify clearly the nature of any concurrent special education or therapeutic programmes and thus it is difficult to establish the natural course of the disorder.

There are reports that refer to the relationship between language disorders and learning disabilities, education, vocational status and social adjustment (Bannatyne, 1971; Johnson, 1968; Johnson and Myklebust, 1967; McGrady and Olson, 1970; Meier, 1971; Rosenthal, 1970).

Hall and Tomblin (1978) reported a follow-up study of 36 language-articulation-impaired children, 13–20 years after having contact with the speech therapy service. They compared 18 language impaired children with 18 who had impaired articulation, on communication status as adults, academic achievement, and level of formal education. The findings indicate that, compared with children who were designated as having an articulation difficulty alone, children who were classified as language impaired had more subsequent communication problems, more academic difficulties particularly in the area of reading and differed in the types of post-secondary education attempted. The description as to whether they were language or articulation impaired was made retrospectively, which may affect the reliability of the study. There is other evidence suggesting that language-disordered pre-school children are at risk for later language, academic and social difficulties (Aram et al., 1984; Aram and Nation, 1980; King et al., 1982; Padget, 1988; Silva et al., 1983; Tallal et al., 1988). Based on the results from these studies, it can be estimated that 40–75% of pre-schoolers with language impairment, will continue to experience difficulties related to this impairment even beyond schooling.

These authors, not surprisingly, call for more appropriate subject details and assessments to be recorded to assist with follow-up studies, which are frequently flawed by poor record keeping in the initial stages of contact.

A study by Tyler (1992), investigated, in more detail, the presenting symptoms of speech and language in order to establish whether the initial diagnosis could be relied upon for future follow-up studies. A detailed study of 12 children between the ages of 21 and 32 months showed that all subjects displayed retarded phonological and language behaviours that were commensurate at their initial evaluation. However, at 1 year follow-up, 25% of the subjects no longer displayed an expressive language delay, and the majority of the subjects were still delayed in development and no longer displayed language and phonological skills that were commensurate. These results point to the need to assess all linguistic behaviours, including phonology, at intake and follow-up, in well-defined prospective studies as it appears that the pattern and relationship between these disorders may change and could be of prognostic significance. The intra-linguistic relationship may well be diagnostic, prognostic and evolutionary (Olswang and Bain, 1991a,b).

Deviance versus delay

The issue of deviance versus delay in phonology and language acquisition has contributed much to the literature. There are those who suggest that certain combinations of characteristics demonstrate deviance whereas others hypothesize that similar characteristics should be regarded as delay. The debate continues regarding the natural course of development of various speech and language processes as the mechanisms of first language acquisition are poorly understood. Theories of language acquisition seek to explain how children learn language within a specific developmental period using similar developmental patterns and normally show similar patterns of error.

Curtis, Katz and Tallal (1992) investigated the issue of delay versus deviance in the language acquisition of language-impaired children (LI). They examined the order of acquisition of a set of linguistic structures, and the relationship between one structure and another in comprehension and production over a 5 year period in a group of 28 language-impaired children and matched normal children.

The results demonstrated a marked similarity between the groups both from the point at which mastery of individual structures was achieved and the overall patterns of acquisition demonstrated. This data suggests that language-impaired children are constructing grammars based on the same laws and principles as those of linguistically normal children and that their linguistic impairments may be principally processing and not representational in nature. These findings are somewhat surprising. The fact of relatively normal grammar acquisition, in the face of neurological and cognitive deficiencies, suggests that the mechanisms of grammar construction in first language acquisition are robust and points to the evolutionary and functional significance of this human faculty. These findings conflict with other studies that report deviance in the language acquisition of LI children. This could be due to the fact that the cohort of this study is more tightly controlled or that the criteria used were somewhat different.

Paul and Jennings (1992) considered the issue of phonological deviance or delay by examining toddlers with slow expressive language development compared with normally speaking age-mates on three global measures of phonological behaviour: the average level of complexity of their syllable structures, the number of different consonant phonemes produced, and the percentage of consonants correctly produced in intelligible utterances. The groups were found to differ significantly on all three variables. Further analyses were made, subdividing the groups to narrower age ranges. These comparisons also revealed differences between late-talking and normal youngsters.

The 28 late talkers showed a delayed rather than deviant pattern, which suggests an intimate connection between speech and language development at this early stage of acquisition. It may be that late talkers have poor phonological skills, reflecting slow oral motor or phonological processing abilities, and that this lag is a primary cause of their slow expressive language development. On the other hand it is possible that phonological skills, in this group, are depressed because the late talkers talk less and get less practice, thus extending and supporting Johnston's (1985) speculations relating to normal development versus delayed development discussed earlier.

Assessment

What to assess?

Identifying developmental language disability has attracted the interest of workers in many different associated professional disciplines and has led to an impressive amount of research during the past 10 years. The majority of studies focus on single aspects of language disorder. For instance, Tallal and Newcombe (1978) claimed that an inability to perceive rapidly changing acoustic stimuli may give rise to poor perception of specific phonemes and also to a disturbance of the temporal sequencing and segmentation of speech. Other researchers have focused on other aspects, e.g. the importance of auditory short-term memory (Bliss and Peterson, 1975). A survey of linguistically orientated and experimental psycholinguistic studies is presented by Johnston (1988) and demonstrates that language impairments have been oversimplified and have many different underlying causes. Assessments usually reflect the hypotheses related to the causes of the particular disorder.

Nettelbladt et al. (1989) present the results from a multi-disciplinary assessment of 10 Swedish children with severe language impairments aged between 4 and 10 years. The children underwent extensive medical examinations and examination by a clinical child psychologist. Neurolinguistic and linguistic analysis was undertaken. The heterogeneity of the patients is described and the authors conclude that detailed case studies are the only way, at present, to elucidate crucial individual differences in language-disordered children. This study underlines the problems that many researchers find in this field. There are few standardized assessments available and commonly in use which would cover the range of disorders that one may find within the subject pool. The amount of subject data used in different research varies, for example, some giving results of detailed audiological examination whereas others may give more information on linguistic analysis but little on hearing acuity.

The paper by Nye and Weems (1991) detailed over 50 different assessments used within the surveys that they reviewed. No study collected information on all the different speech and language features of the subject. It is possible that different combinations of phonological disorders and language impairments, may identify different sub-groups. Furthermore, detailing of specific neurological findings, such as minimal coordination difficulties and responsivity, could again assist in identifying commonalities. The effects of social, psychological and environmental aspects, which may affect not only language development, but also treatment outcome, have only been addressed in a few studies.

In addition to all the factors that need to be assessed, as they may affect the different type of disorder and its outcome to therapy, we also have to consider the speech and language sample itself. More researchers have become concerned about the limitations of standardized assessment procedures, particularly for very young children, and whilst these may be useful for documenting global change in behaviour, they may not be the best tools for obtaining frequent repeated measurements regarding the effects of intervention. Consequently, speech and language therapists have been turning more to conversational sampling to quantify children's performance of specific language behaviours over time. But language sampling is not as straightforward a task as it may seem; the complexity lies in the need to obtain an adequate sample of the child's language over time to determine whether growth has occurred.

Bain, Olswang and Johnson (1992) compared the outcomes of two methods of sampling speech, one in free play and another in a structured activity. The results of the investigation suggested that the children were able to demonstrate a better outcome to treatment in a free play situation than if they had been assessed in the structured situation alone. The free play situation in the study was structured in that enough materials were provided to ensure opportunities for language behaviours of interest to be stimulated and it appears that this could be a practical way of providing supporting material to assess a child's progress.

Masterson and Kamhi (1991) comment that:

> One goal of language sampling is to determine a child's competence regarding use of advanced sentence structures and the child must be provided with tasks that will increase the probability of the use of such structures. For exam-

ple, we found that the absence of pictures and props resulted in the use of more compound sentence structures.

The findings of this study suggest that using pictures and objects may, in fact, be counter productive in obtaining optimal language production.

Developing this theme further, Hansson and Nettelbladt (1990) considered the interactional aspects of language that may be missed in the usual linguistic or standardized speech and language assessments. They detailed a method of audio-taping verbal interactions between child and clinician talking about pictures, games and drawings. The method was tried on four children and demonstrated that dialogue information could be transcribed. This, they speculated, could improve the ability to diagnose and carry out therapy as it gives more information regarding the child's strategies in conversation and how the partner's communicative style can influence the child.

Treatment Efficacy

The profession of speech and language therapy has only relatively recently tried to address the difficult area of documenting the effectiveness of treatment with this client group (Olswang, 1990). The profession has strived to move from an intuitive artistic understanding of the concepts of interaction, to a more considered and scientific approach, which necessitates the empirical demonstration of effective clinical procedures, testing the theoretical underpinning of treatment, and determining the validity and utility of assessments (Damico, 1988; Ringel *et al.*, 1984).

Reviewing the recent literature has identified several different approaches to the efficacy question. There are a group of studies examining what has happened to clients who have received speech and language therapy. Other studies have tested different specific treatment programmes with small numbers of individual children using single case studies and multiple baseline techniques to monitor change. A third approach has concentrated on the comparison of different deliveries of therapy, i.e. therapists versus parents or teachers, to establish the cost effectiveness/ effectiveness of different delivery modes.

Retrospective follow-up studies

In 1985, Paul Weiner published a thoughtful summary of 17 follow-up studies of children with speech and/or language problems. Follow-up studies should be seen as a valuable source of information to help with greater understanding of the underlying disorders and to assist with prediction. However, there are methodological problems in retrospective studies of this type. These include the changing paradigms over time, changing definitions, loss to follow-up, lack of initial subject detail, and the possibility of bias. Despite this there appears to be some common themes in the findings of follow-up studies.

Huntley *et al.* (1988) followed up 119 children referred for speech and language therapy because of severe language delay. The first follow-up showed that a higher percentage (30%) of 20 children who were referred but had not received treatment made a poor outcome. All those receiving treatment showed considerable improvement and, in a follow-up 5 years later, of 63 of the original cohort, this was maintained, although the gains were smaller than was measured at the intervention period.

Ripley (1986) reviewed 120 children, seen at a special residential unit for specific speech and language disorders between 1979 and 1985. There were 12 receptive dysphasics, 21 expressive dysphasics, 57 with specific language delay and 30 with articulation disorders. The authors found that 35.8% of children went to normal schools once discharged and all the individuals were noted as showing 'significant gains'.

Shriberg and Kwiatkowski (1988) followed up 36 children who had received pre-school speech and language therapy for phonological disorders. Their findings are more detailed than the previous studies and show that this cohort was more severely affected than those of some other studies. However, it is similar to other studies in that a high proportion continued to need extended specific education. Children who had only phonological difficulties required less special education and services than those initially demonstrating more complex problems, i.e. combined speech and language impairments. Interestingly, the severity of the phonological problem and intelligibility were not good predictors.

These findings are amplified by a smaller study undertaken by Scarborough and Dobrich (1990), which followed up four subjects from the age of 2.5–5 years who had early language impairment showing severe and broad impairments in syntactic, phonological and lexical production. The findings were compared with 12 controls who had no speech and language impairment but were of similar age. Over time the deficits became milder and more selective, thus a diffuse problem became more specific as the children became older and, by 60 months, three had normal speech and language. However, 3 years later, three of the cohort were found to have reading problems. The relationship between early speech and language disorders and later specific educational/social difficulties has been referred to in many papers. It is possibly one of the reasons why a child studied by Damico (1988), demonstrated a strange language development history. This child, who was 12 years old, had received detailed speech and language therapy and was discharged, reportedly having achieved acceptable speech and language production. However, a later review found that the child had a specific language disorders that were causing problems within the school and home setting. Damico calls for long-term follow-up of children who have had marked speech and language disorders early in life, as it is possible that the changing context and the greater demands placed on the child later will reveal further difficulties which are not apparent when the child enters school. This calls into question the issue of what is a successful outcome to therapy.

Another interesting issue is raised. As discussed earlier, classification is essential if one is to be able to compare studies and generalize results. This is also important when considering the theoretical principles underlying language breakdown and its therapy. If, as these studies demonstrate, the nature of the relationship between the different components of speech and language varies over time then classification systems have to be able to reflect this change appropriately.

Efficacy of different modes of therapy delivery

Several studies have looked at using parents as an alternative or additional therapy source. These papers considered efficacy relating to the mode of delivery of therapy and in some instances have looked at the cost-effectiveness of these.

Fey *et al.* (1993) studied 30 pre-school children with language impairment particularly related to poor grammatical development. Their ages were between 3 years 8 months and 5 years 10 months. They were allocated to having therapy at a clinic with speech and language therapists, or with the parents who were trained by therapists. The third group were delayed in the receipt of treatment and served as a control. The treatment was carried out over 4 months and the language samples were elicited during play. The children treated by therapists and those treated by parents improved. The therapists' gains were more consistent, i.e. more aspects of the language disorder improved and there was less variability. The children who had deferred treatment did not show any gains during the same period. This paper has a good description of therapy but gives the same warning as other similar studies, that the parents required a significant input from the therapist in order to train them. However, the length of time for professional input to the parent group was approximately 50% less than for the group treated by the therapist alone.

Similarly, Ruscello *et al.* (1993) monitored the changes in 12 pre-school children, aged between 4 years 1 month and 5 years 8 months, with phonological process errors who were randomly assigned to one of two treatments that differed in relation to service delivery. The first group received treatment that was administered exclusively by the clinician, the second group received a combination that included clinician-administered treatment and parent-administered instruction, the latter being supported with the Speech Viewer computer system. Both groups received 16 lessons over 8 weeks and both showed significant improvement with no significant difference between the groups.

A carefully designed study, presented in thesis form in 1991 by Lancaster, examined 15 children with phonological problems who were randomly assigned to one of three groups. One group received individual weekly therapy from a speech and language therapist, in the second group, therapy was delivered by their parents following training by a speech and language therapist, the third group were assessed and their treatment deferred. The two treatment groups made significantly more improvement than the untreated group and again there was no significant difference between the parental and the therapist delivery.

The costing implications regarding parents taking more responsibility for therapy delivery was considered in a study of 40 pre-school speech-disordered children who were 'moderately disordered' and were assigned (not randomly) to having clinic-based therapy versus a parental programme (Eiserman et al., 1990). They received once-a-week treatment over a protracted period. Children in the groups, at base line, were found to be comparable on most of the significant aspects of medical, social, and speech history. There was no significant difference on post-test speech and language therapy tasks between those treated by the parents and those by the therapists. However, the parental group did show a trend to more improvement on articulation tasks. The amount of training given to the mothers was significant and this led to no meaningful cost benefit of delivering therapy in this way. The authors warned, that the study group was relatively middle class, with none of the mothers going out to work.

One year later, the children were followed up (Eiserman et al., 1992) and it was established that there was no significant difference in speech and general developmental measures between the two groups but the personal social skills and adaptive behaviour showed a trend towards a better outcome for the parental treated group. The difference in articulation in the parental treated group noted after the first study was no longer apparent. These authors point to the need for further research about the long-term benefits of parents who have been trained to work with their child and the extent to which parents are able to generalize their training to working with other children in their family or to other educational areas.

Other studies indicating the value of a structured approach to using mothers as agents include Weistuch and Byers Brown (1987); Masterson (1993); Newman and Elks (1988). Peers were found to be of assistance by Goldstein and Strain (1988).

A paper by Dodd and Barker (1990) gives less detailed information but addresses a similar and interesting question in two studies in children with phonological disorders. The first looks at the outcome of five children when the parents acted as the main agents of therapy, the second study with six slightly older children, examined the outcome when teachers were the primary agents of therapy. The outcome showed that three of the children in the parental group did not require further therapy whereas all of those in the teachers' group required continued therapy. Considerable time was spent in training the teachers and there were fewer positive results from this group presumably because their energies were dissipated over a larger number of children.

Specific speech and language therapy approaches for phonological disorders

Therapists, when planning treatment for severely disordered children, have to consider which targets would be most appropriate. The literature has proposed that stimulability is a factor that should be considered, i.e. if a sound can be stimulated it is more likely to be able to be achieved within treatment and generalized to spontaneous speech.

Some schools of thought consider stimulability as a global ability of the child rather than an attribute specific to the phoneme. A study by Powell, Elbert and Dinnsen (1991) examined whether more stimulable targets were achievable in therapy and would be generalizable and also the question of whether it was a specific or global attribute. Six children, aged between 4 years 11 months and 5 years 6 months, who demonstrated phonological disorders, were subjects in a multiple baseline single subject design. Three hundred and six items were chosen as probes. All children were taught /r/ and one other sound which was not within their repertoire. Production of stimulable sounds tended to improve regardless of the treatment target, and generalized but nonstimulable sounds did not generalize and it was speculated that they would require direct therapy.

The use of minimal pairs as a method of facilitating improved articulatory performance has been documented for the past 20 years. Weiner (1981), was one of the first to test this approach in a multi-response base line procedure with two 4-year-old children with phonological impairment. The programme of therapy, which was over 14 sessions, demonstrated that minimal pair contrastive therapy, which is extremely well described within this paper, led to improvement and generalization to non-treated words in both subjects. The question as to whether minimal or maximal pair therapy should be used did not arise until later. Maximal pair therapy requires the therapist to use words in treatment showing many distinctive features. Gierut (1990) reported three children in a multiple baseline study comparing minimal/maximal pair therapy. Maximal pair therapy was found to be of value for some sounds and the author speculates that a treatment programme starting with multiple/maximal distinctions, leading to multiple distinctions and then minimal distinctions, would be more efficacious than instantly starting with minimal distinctive pairs. The speculation goes beyond that supported by the data but it is an interesting concept that would be worthy of further investigation.

A further common principle in therapy has been that of providing the correct model for a child immediately after he or she makes an error, in order to facilitate learning. The child is not directly corrected. This method (correct model/naturalistic conversation training/direct conversation therapy) has been used by Camarata (1993) with children with both phonological and language impairments. For the former, the author used a multiple baseline design with two children who had 36 sessions of treatment. Base lines prior to the approach showed no progress in the target behaviours before treatment commenced. During treatment the correct model was given after the child said the word incorrectly and this was termed 'naturalistic conversation training'. Both children improved and generalized. The author suggests that what they required was an increased number of relevant and immediate models.

Many different technological supports, to assist with the treatment of phonological disorders, have been described. Visual representation of sound, bio-feedback and intraoral appliances have been cited in the literature. Few have been tested for their efficacy. An exception to this has been the testing of an intraoral appliance which was devised to facilitate the correction of the production of /r/ sound (Clark et al., 1993). This device was evaluated in a study of 36 children, aged between 8 and 12 years old, who had been referred because of difficulty in producing the phoneme /r/. Four treatment groups were formed and the groups were randomly allocated to a treatment period of 6 weeks with or without the appliance and with or without auditory monitoring to assist. There were statistically better results for the children who had the appliance with or without auditory monitoring. However, the best spontaneous speech results were achieved in the group who had the combination of the auditory model and the appliance.

A seminal review of 63 published reports in which the effectiveness of treatment of articulation or phonological disorders was evaluated (Sommers et al., 1992), showed that the designs most frequently used were case study (13), multiple baseline across behaviours (9), withdrawal and reversal design (7), and independent group and random assignment (60). Of 30 research designs, described by Doehring (1988), only 15 were used in the research reviewed. Of the 63 articles, 33 were published in the 1970s and demonstrated limitations: frequent absence of descriptive information about subjects; lack of detail regarding duration and extent of treatment; frequent absence of a follow-up phase; very small numbers of subjects in the group studies; lack of detail regarding random selection of subjects; lack of reliability information; and failure to state dependant variables.

Of 30 research reports reviewed from the 1980s, 23 were of a single subject design. However, there continued to be a lack of descriptive information about subjects and frequently the extent and duration of treatment was sparsely reported. Only 6 of the 30 had a follow-up phase and reported randomization of subject selection. The authors conclude that whilst positive changes have occurred in the research design and methodology from the 1970s into the 1980s a number of negative research practices still continue.

Sommers, Logston and Wright (1992) quite rightly advocate neither more nor less of each type of research, but the importance of conducting **better** research:

> It is also apparent that 63 research reports across 2 decades of publications in the 4 major journals that contain most of the literature does not reflect the need for efficacy data related to articulation and phonological disorders, because the prevalence of these disorders is high in the case loads of many practitioners. For many important clinical decisions that occur routinely, estimations of efficacy of treatment data are needed that are based upon both comprehensive single subject designs and more powerful designs that provide reliable replication. It is regrettable that published information in the 1980s was no stronger in meeting these needs, and in some ways, was actually weaker in doing so.

Specific speech and language therapy for language impairment

Natural maturational improvement may confound investigations into the effectiveness of speech and language therapy for both phonological and language disorders. As a practical matter:

> 'It is very difficult to demonstrate long term effects for preschool interventions for specific language delays given the very high rates of spontaneous resolution for all forms of language delays that have previously been documented as occurring throughout the preschool period' (Whitehurst and Fischel, 1994).

Telleen and Wren (1985), acknowledging this problem, devised a study investigating the effectiveness of teaching prepositions to language-delayed pre-schoolers. Twenty-five children between the ages of 3.0 and 5.6 years received therapy over a 5 month period and showed a significant gain in preposition comprehension. Their progress was compared with that of 51 normal pre-school children aged between 2.11 and 5.10 years who were observed at similar intervals to establish the process of maturation. The authors conclude that the specific teaching of prepositions had an effect on the language-impaired group beyond that of maturation.

Efficacy studies, focused on word-finding intervention in children, are sparse; those that have been conducted have contrasted elaboration with retrieval treatment procedures to enhance children's word-finding skills. Elaboration treatment provides children with a richer knowledge of the target word to assist their retrieval. Retrieval treatment teaches children to use phonemic, locative and category retrieval cues to enhance their word-finding skills. Contrasting these treatment procedures, McGregor and Leonard (1989), studying children with both language comprehension problems and word-finding difficulties, indicated that a word-finding treatment that combined both techniques was the most effective as measured by increased accuracy on picture naming. Similarly, Rubin, Rotella and Schwartz (1988), reported improvement in picture-naming performance of third-graders with age appropriate language skills after training that combined both elaborative and retrieval approaches.

Wing (1990) reported somewhat different results. The effects of three treatment programmes were compared: a semantic treatment to improve elaboration and organization of the semantic lexicon; a phonological treatment to increase meta-linguistic awareness of the phonological structure; a perceptual imagery treatment that provided auditory and visual imagery cues. The author noted that subjects receiving the phonological and imagery treatments improved significantly in retrieving untrained targets whereas the semantic treatment group made no significant improvement. Whilst the results from all these investigations indicate that specific intervention can improve word-finding skills in children they conflict regarding the appropriateness of the different techniques used. Some authors differ as to what they identify as representative of these remedial approaches. German (1992) indicates that rhyming techniques are referred to as elaboration training in one investigation (McGregor and Leonard, 1989) and as a phonological treatment in another study (Wing, 1990).

Comparison of two treatment methods was used by Haynes (1992), not only to examine the efficacy of the treatment but also to question the underlying problem in an apparently similar defect exhibited by two boys aged 10 and 11 years. Thirty-two target words were selected, some to be treated by elaboration and some by definition. One child progressed in both conditions and one child showed no progress in either. The study shows a number of weaknesses that were acknowledged by the author and there is an apparent lack of any statistical information. However, it is an important paper as it tests issues of classification by looking at responses to specific treatment programmes.

One aspect of language therapy that causes difficulty to therapists is to keep a track of the therapy goals. Mineo and Goldstein (1990) tested the effectiveness of a matrix training programme, which is a simple method of detailing the language to be targeted. A multiple base-line design was used with four language-delayed pre-school children, aged between 2 years 7 months and 4 years 11 months, in a structured programme to facilitate reception and expressive language. All subjects demonstrated no gains on baseline but noticeable gains during the treatment period, particularly expressively, with increase in length of utterances. Generalization was also noticed in all subjects.

A direct therapeutic approach can be compared with an indirect one. Camarata and Nelson (1992) compared indirect conversation therapy with a directly elicited imitation approach with four language-impaired children aged between 4 years 9 months and 5 years 11 months. The chosen targets, all absent from the original speech sample, were randomly assigned to treatment by one of these two approaches. All four subjects improved. Those facilitated by the conversational therapy showed better results but the imitation therapy facilitated some specific acquisitions.

Some of the terms used to describe different therapy programmes are, in themselves, confusing. It is not clear whether the work by Weismer and Branch (1989), comparing modelling alone with modelling with evoked production, is similar to the work described in the previous study. It appears that there are fundamental differences but it is likely that there are also similarities.

There are different views as to whether generalization is promoted more by a child being the passive recipient of a positively reinforcing environment which is deemed by its nature to influence behaviour or whether a more active participation has better effect. In reality, it is likely that the abilities, age and deficits of children may lead them to benefit or not from one or other of these particular approaches. Unfortunately, our knowledge for categorizing individual children does not assist us in examining which approach is most suitable for which children (Connell, 1987; Howell and Dean, 1987).

Therapy for children with more than one disorder

The co-occurrence of phonological and language disorders has been acknowledged for some time. It has been estimated that 75–80% of children with phonological disorders have associated language involvement (Shriberg et al., 1986). Thus, many children require attention to both aspects and there is debate about which treatment should be instigated first. Wing (1990) addresses the close association of phonological and language impairment in a study of two groups of 6-year-old language-impaired children, receiving 30 treatments over a 10 week period. The aim of the study was to contrast the effects of two treatment programmes on generalization to untrained words in a picture-naming task. The treatment programmes were a traditional semantic association approach, using techniques involving categorization, association, part, whole, etc and a programme focused on phonological and perceptual components of retrieval process, including picture naming, segmentation, and training of visual and auditory memory. The subjects receiving the phonological and perceptual treatment improved significantly in naming untrained pictures, but the semantic treatment group made no significant improvement. The author hypothesizes that the results are related to Wolf's multi-staged model (1982) of retrieval process, as the perceptual and phonological processes described in Wolf's model may have been improved by imagery and segmentation treatment.

Tyler and Waterson (1991), examined 12 children aged between 3 years 7 months and 5 years 7 months, who were matched at baseline with phonological and language impairment, who were 1 year below their chronological age in expressive language. Subjects were matched and then randomly assigned to receiving treatment, emphasizing either phonological intervention, or language intervention. They had two sessions of therapy per week for 6 weeks. Those treated with phonological approach improved both in language and phonology, whilst the language group improved only on language and regressed on phonology. There are marked implications of this study and further research is justifiably called for by the authors.

Another group of children with multifactorial difficulties are those who stutter and exhibit other speech, voice and language problems (Nippold 1990). It is unclear whether the concomitant problems should be ignored, treated prior to the stammer, following the stammer, or with the stammer. Conture, Louko, and Edwards (1993) addressed this issue in a preliminary study. They followed up two groups of children aged about 6 years. One group had stammering and phonological problems and one group demonstrated fluency disorders only. Both groups had weekly group therapy over a 12 month period aimed either at a stammering and phonology programme or at stammering alone. Both groups showed considerable improvement and the authors suggest that you can treat the two disorders simultaneously without having a negative affect upon the fluency.

Conclusion

The studies cited here all give information that assists with the examination of the efficacy of speech and language therapy for children with speech and language disorders. Follow-up studies suggest that children with speech and language impairments may well have diffuse complex problems initially and that these will evolve to more specific difficulties later in life. There appears to be a strong association between early speech and language problems and later difficulties with certain educational tasks such as reading.

There is strong evidence that a number of children with speech and language disorders at an early age (2 years old) will grow out of their difficulties and whilst they may benefit from speech and language therapy in the short term, and their recovery may be expedited, in the long term there may not be any difference between this group and similar children not receiving therapy. What is difficult for researchers and practitioners is to identify those children who have disorders that indicate a broader range of underlying difficulties which will not be resolved or may lead to a different spectrum of difficulties in later life. It is essential that the research addresses the issue of identifying the criteria that will indicate those children who will grow out of their problems and those who have factors that may lead to long-term difficulties.

The specific speech and language therapy techniques that have been tested have mostly been found to be efficacious, but there are still major issues that need to addressed. There are fundamental problems regarding the terminology and classification of speech and language disorders in children. This relates not only to the description of the disorders themselves but also to the therapeutic programmes and theoretical underpinnings. Many similar concepts and issues are termed differently by different authors.

Olswang and Bain (1991a,b) recommend a data-based approach for determining when a child with language disorders can benefit from intervention. Profiling, dynamic assessment and tracking are the procedures they recommend for helping the speech and language pathologist to determine when a child can benefit from intervention. There appears to be no doubt not only that better accessible data could improve organization of clinical services but also that the field could benefit from more controlled retrospective studies. But for these to be achieved there is an urgent requirement for a core information set, which is agreed, so that researchers in the field can gather similar information on clients, thus allowing studies to be compared and information to be pooled.

The issue regarding delivery of therapy has been addressed quite convincingly. Nearly all the studies showed that parents can be used productively to assist in delivering therapy. Obviously there are some specific disorders or some particular parents whose attitudes or abilities would not necessarily lend themselves to this approach. However, despite the research evidence, the active promotion of parental involvement in therapy is underdeveloped. Research to date highlights that parental and teacher involvement requires a heavy input from the speech and language therapist.

Bain and Dollaghan (1991) suggest, that for a change to be considered clinically significant it must be:

- The result of treatment rather than from maturation.
- Real as opposed to random.
- Important rather than trivial.

These appear to be very logical but are much harder in reality to implement. The single subject design using multiple base line helps in overcoming some of the concerns. Additionally, larger cohorts with periods of pre-treatment observation would also assist. There should also be more attention to studies observing the natural history of the patterns of different disorders.

Another issue concerns the amount and quality of research in this field. Given that approximately 70% of the speech and language therapy resource in the UK is spent on children with speech and language difficulties, the amount of research is inadequate. Additionally there appear to be very few good detailed follow-up studies with large cohorts. This is despite the fact that virtually every speech and language therapy clinic has access to a large amount of clinical data. There must be ways of improving our access to data and the way in which we store it so that we can benefit from the clinical information over time.

References

Adams C and Bishop DVM (1989). Conversational characteristics of children with semantic-pragmatic disorder I: Structure, turn taking, repairs and cohesion. British Journal of Disorders of Communication 14: 211–239.

Aram DM, Ekelman BL and Nation JE (1984). Pre-schoolers with language disorders: Ten years later. Journal of Speech and Hearing Research 27: 232–244.

Aram DM and Nation JE (1980). Pre-school language disorders and subsequent language and academic difficulties. Journal of Communication Disorders 13: 159–170.

Bain BA and Dollaghan C (1991). Clinical forum: Treatment efficacy; the notion of clinically significant change. Language, Speech and Hearing Services in Schools 22: 264–270.

Bain B, Olswang LB and Johnson GA (1992). Language sampling for repeated measures with language impaired pre-Schoolers: Comparison of two procedures. Topics in Language Disorders 12(2): 13–27.

Bannatyne A (1971). Language reading and learning disabilities. Springfield, IL Charles C Thomas.

Bishop DVM and Adams C (1989). Conversational characteristics of children with semantic-pragmatic disorders II: What features led to a judgement of inappropriatcy? British Journal of Disorders of Communication 24: 241–263.

Bishop DVM and Adams C (1992). Comprehension of problem children with specific language impairment: Literal and inference meaning. Journal of Speech and Hearing Research 35: 119–130.

Bishop DVM and Edmundson A (1987). Specific language impairment as a maturational lag: Evidence from longitudinal data on language and motor development. Developmental Medicine and Child Neurology 19: 442–449.

Bliss LS and Peterson DM (1975). Performance of aphasic and non aphasic children on a sentence repetition task. Journal of Communication Disorders 8: 207–212.

British Telecom. Speakwatch Campaign Survey (1994). Available from Paragon Communications: Wardour Street, London.

Butler NR, Peckham C and Sheridan M. (1973). Speech defects in children aged 7 years: A national study. British Medical Journal 3: 255–257.

Camarata (1993). The application of naturalistic conversation training to speech production in children with speech disabilities. Journal of Applied Behaviour Analysis 26: 173–182.

Camarata SM and Nelson KE (1992). Treatment efficiency as a function of target selection in the remediation of child language disorders. Clinical Linguistics and Phonetics 6(3): 167–178.

Clark CE, Schwarz IE and Blakeley RW (1993). The removable R-appliance as a practice device to facilitate correct production of /r/. American Journal of Speech Language Pathology 2:84–92.

Connell P (1987). An effect of modelling and imitation teaching procedures on children with and without specific language impairment. Journal of Speech and Hearing Research 30: 105–113.

Conture EG, Louko LJ and Edwards ML (1993). Simultaneously treating stuttering and disordered phonology in children: Experimental treatment preliminary findings. American Journal of Speech Language Pathology 2: 71–81.

Curtis S, Katz W and Tallal P (1992). Delay versus deviance in the language acquisition of language impaired children. Journal of Speech and Hearing Research 35: 373–383.

Damico JS (1988). The lack of efficacy in language therapy: A case study. Language, Speech and Hearing Services in Schools 19: 41–50.

Dodd B and Barker R (1990). The efficacy of utilizing parents and teachers as agents of therapy for children with phonological disorders. Australian Journal of Human Communication Disorders 18(1): 29–44.

Doehring DG (1988). Research Strategies in Human Communication Disorders. Boston: Littlebrown.

Eiserman WD, McCoun M and Escobar C (1990). A cost effectiveness analysis of two alternative programme models for serving speech disordered pre-schoolers. Journal of Early Intervention 14(4): 297–317.

Eiserman WD, Weber C and McCoun M (1992). Two alternative programme models for serving speech disordered preschoolers: A second year follow-up. Journal of Communication Disorders 25: 77–106.

Enderby PM and Davies P (1989). Communication disorders: Planning a service to meet the needs. British Journal of Disorders of Communication 24: 301–331.

Fey ME, Cleave PL, Long SH and Hughes DL (1993). Two approaches to the facilitation of grammar in children with language impairment: An experimental evaluation. Journal of Speech and Hearing Research 36: 141–157.

German DJ (1992). Word intervention for children and adolescents. Topics in Language Disorders 13(1): 33–50.

Gierut SA (1990). Differential learning of phonological oppositions. Journal of Speech and Hearing Research 33: 540–549.

Goldstein H and Strain P (1988). Peers as communication intervention agents: Some new strategies and research findings. Topics in Language Disorders 1: 44–57.

Hall PK and Tomblin JB (1978). A follow-up study of children with articulation and language disorders. Journal of Speech and Hearing Disorders 43: 227–241.

Hansson K and Nettelbladt U (1990). The verbal interaction of Swedish language disordered pre-school children. Clinical Linguistics and Phonetics 4(1): 39–48.

Haynes C (1992). Vocabulary deficit-one problem or many? Child language teaching and therapy 8(1): 2–17.

Heltman HJ (1936). Re-education techniques and speech correction. Journal of Speech Disorders 284–289.

Howell J and Dean E (1987). I think that's a noisy sound: Reflection and learning in the therapeutic situation. Child Language, Teaching and Therapy 3: 259–266.

Huntley RMC, Holt KS, Butterfill A and Latham C (1988). A follow-up study of a language intervention programme. British Journal of Disorders of Communication 23: 127–140.

Ingram TT (1972). Classification of speech and language disorders in young children. In: Rutter M and Martin J (Eds) The Child with Delayed Speech. London: Spastics International Medicine.

Johnson DJ (1968). The language continuum. Bulletin of Orton Society 28: 1–11.

Johnson DJ and Myklebust HR (1967). Learning Disabilities: Educational Principles. New York: Grune and Stratton.

Johnson W (1967). Speech Handicapped School Children. 3rd Edition. New York: Harper Row.

Johnston JR (1985). Fit, focus and functionality. Child Language Teaching and Therapy 1(2): 125–134.

Johnston J (1988). Generalization: the nature of change. Language Speech and Hearing Services in Schools 19: 314–327.

King R, Jones D and Lasky E (1982). In retrospect: A fifteen year follow-up of speech and language disordered children. Language Speech and Hearing Services in School 13: 24–32.

Lancaster G (1991). The Effectiveness of Parent Administered Input Training for Children with Phonological Disorders. MSc thesis, City University, London.

Masterson JJ (1993) Classroom based phonological intervention. AJSLP 5–9.

Masterson JJ and Kamhi AG (1991). The effects of sampling conditions on sentence production in normal, reading disabled and language learning disabled children. Journal of Speech and Hearing Research 34: 549–559.

McGrady HJ and Olson DA (1970). Visual and auditory learning processes in normal children and children with learning disabilities. Exceptional Children 36: 581–589.

McGregor KK and Leonard LB (1989). Facilitating word finding skills of language impaired children. Journal of Speech and Hearing Disorders 54: 141–147.

Meier JH (1971). Prevalence and characteristics of learning disabilities found in second grade children. Journal of Learning Disabilities 4: 1–16.

Mineo BA and Goldstein H (1990). Generalised learning of receptive and expressive action object responses by language delayed pre-schoolers. Journal of Speech and Hearing Disorders 55: 665–678.

Morley ME (1972). The Development and Disorders of Speech in Childhood, 3rd Edition. Edinburgh: Churchill Livingstone.

Nettelbladt U, Sahlen B, Ors M and Johannesson P (1989). A multi-disciplinary assessment of children with severe language disorder. Clinical Linguistics and Phonetics 3(4): 313 -346.

Newman and Elks (1988). Working together: A joint phonology and reading programme. Child Language Teaching and Therapy 4: 297–310.

Nippold M (1990). Concomitant speech language disorders in stuttering children: A critique of the literature. Journal of Speech Hearing and Disorders 55: 51–60.

Nye C and Weems L (1991). Identification criteria for children with language disorders. Hearsay 6(1): 34–39.

Olswang LB (1990). Treatment efficacy research: A path to quality assurance. ASHA 32: 45 -47.

Olswang LB and Bain BA (1991a). Clinical forum: Treatment of efficacy; when to recommend intervention. Language, Speech and Hearing Services in Schools 22: 255–263.

Olswang LB and Bain BA (1991b). Intervention issues for toddlers with specific language impairments. Topics in Language Disorders 11: 69–86.

Padget SY (1988). Speech and language impaired three and four year olds: A five year follow-up study. In: Masland RL and Masland MW (Eds) Pre-School Prevention of Reading Failure. Parkton, MD: York Press.

Paul R and Jennings P (1992). Phonological behaviour in toddlers with slow expressive language development. Journal of Speech and Hearing Research 35: 99–107.

Peckham CS (1973). Speech defects in a national sample of children aged 7 years. British Journal of Disorders of Communication 8: 2–8.

Powell TW, Elbert M and Dinnsen DA (1991). Stimulability as a factor in the phonological generalization of mis-articulating pre-school children. Journal of Speech and Hearing Research 34: 1318–1328.

Quirk R (1972). Speech Therapy Services. London: HMSO.

Ringel RL, Trachtman LE and Prutting CA (1984). The science in human communication sciences. ASHA 26: 33–37.

Ripley K (1986). The Moor House School Remedial Programme: An evaluation. Child Language Teaching and Therapy 2(3): 282–299.

Rosenthal JH (1970). A preliminary psycholinguistic study of children with learning disabilities. Journal of Learning Disabilities 3: 391–395.

Rubin H, Rotella T and Schwartz L (1988). The effect of phonological analysis training on naming performance. Unpublished Manuscript. (Referred to in German 1992.)

Ruscello DM, Cartwright LR, Haines KB and Shuster LI (1993). Use of different service models for children with phonological disorders. Journal of Communication Disorders 26: 193–203.

Scarborough HS and Dobrich W (1990). Development of children with early language delay. Journal of Speech and Hearing Research 33: 70–83.

Shriberg LD, Kwiatkowski J, Best S, Hengst J and Terselic-Weber B (1986). Characteristics of children with phonologic disorders of unknown origin. Journal of Speech and Hearing Disorders 51: 140–161.

Shriberg LD and Kwiatkowski J (1988). A follow-up study of children with phonologic disorders of unknown origin. Journal of Speech and Hearing Disorders 53: 144–155.

Silva P, McGhee R and Williams S (1987). Developmental language delay from 3 to 7 years and its significance for low intelligence and reading difficulties at age 7. Developmental Medicine and Child Neurology 25(6): 783–793.

Snow C, Midkiff-Borunda MS, Small A and Proctor A (1984). Therapy as social interaction: analyzing the contexts for language remediation. Topics in Language Disorders 4(3): 72–85.

Sommers RK, Logston BS and Wright JM (1992). A review and critical analysis of treatment research related to articulation and phonological disorders. Journal of Communication Disorders 25: 3–22.

Stark R and Tallal P (1981). Selection of children with specific language deficits. Journal of Speech and Hearing Disorders 46: 161–180.

Tallal P, Curtiss S and Kaplan R (1988). The San Diego Longitudinal Study: Evaluating the outcomes of pre-school impairment in language development. In: Gerber S and Mencher G (Eds) International Perspectives in Communication Disorders. Washington DC: Gallndet University Press, 86–126.

Tallal P and Newcombe F (1978). Impairment of auditory perception and language comprehension in dysphasia. Brain and Language 5: 13–24.

Telleen S and Wren C (1985). Acquisition of prepositions in language-delayed pre-schoolers: Is intervention effective? British Journal of Disorders of Communication 20: 301–309.

Tyler AA (1992). Profiles of a relationship between phonology and language in late talkers. Child Language Teaching and Therapy 8: 246–264.

Tyler AA and Waterson KH (1991). Effects of phonological versus language intervention in pre-schoolers with both phonological and language impairment. Child Language Teaching and Therapy 7(2): 141–160.

Weiner F (1981). Treatment of phonological disability using the method of meaningful minimal contrast: Two case studies. Journal of Speech and Hearing Disorders 46: 97 -103.

Weiner P (1985). The value of follow-up studies. Topics in Language Disorders 5: 78 - 92.

Weismer SE and Branch J (1989). Modelling versus modelling plus evoked production training: A comparison of two language intervention methods. Journal of Speech and Hearing Disorders 54: 269–281.

Weistuch L and Byers Brown B (1987). Motherese as therapy; a programme and its dissemination. Child Language Teaching and Therapy 3(1): 57–70.

Whitehurst GJ and Fischel JE (1994). Practitioner review: Early developmental language delay: what, if anything, should the clinician do about it? Journal of Child Psychology and Psychiatry 35(4): 613–648.

Wing CS (1990). A preliminary investigation of generalisation to untrained words following two treatments of children's word-finding problems. Language Speech and Hearing Services in Schools 21: 151–156.

Wolf M (1982). The word-retrieval process and reading in children and aphasics. In: Nelson K (Ed.) Children's Language 3: 437–493.

Chapter 4
Cleft Palate

Introduction

Although cleft lip and cleft palate are frequently discussed together there is good embryological and genetic evidence that cleft palate is developmentally and genetically different from cleft lip (Fraser, 1970). Cleft palate (i.e. without cleft of lip) is less frequent than cleft lip (with or without cleft palate) and there is much less genetic data available. The main causes of cleft palate are generally thought to be related to major mutant genes, chromosomal abnormalities, environmental factors, e.g. pollutants, and a combination of these and other factors. It is thought that the proportion of multi-factorial cases may be smaller than for cleft lip (Spriestersbach *et al.*, 1973). Cleft lip and/or palate are frequently a part of a syndrome of defects where the patient has associated groups of impairments. Over 400 known syndromes involve clefts of the lip or palate with more than a third of these caused by major mutant genes and some resulting from recognized chromosomal aberrations.

McWilliams and Matthews (1979) related types of congenital abnormalities to cleft type in a study of 226 subjects. They found that 18% of the subjects with isolated palatal clefts had some type of syndrome, whereas none of the subjects with complete clefts of the lip and palate had an identifiable syndrome. Among the children who had other associated defects, 70% of those with isolated palatal clefts had skeletal deformities, 36% had defects of the urinary/genital system, and gastro-intestinal defects were found in 31%.

Prevalence

A conservative estimate of the incidence appears to be approximately 1 in every 600 live births although there are some indications that the rate is different in some parts of the world, e.g. 1 in 462 live births in Finland (Jenson *et al.*, 1988). This estimate does not include certain minimal expressions of the defect such as a bifid uvula or submucous clefts. Bifid uvula may have an incidence rate of 1 in 80 caucasians (Gorlin *et al.*, 1976) whereas submucous cleft is an abnormality which occurs in about 1 in 1200 births (Moss *et al.*, 1988). There are tentative indications that the rate of occurrence of cleft lip and/or cleft palate may be higher than it was. This may be the result of better medical treatment allowing more pregnancies to come to term and more high-risk infants surviving and thriving. Additionally, more adults with cleft palate are able to live a normal life, producing children and thus increasing the size of the genetic pool that carries the cleft trait (McWilliams *et al.*, 1990). Although it is well established that cleft lip, with or without cleft palate, occurs about twice as often in males as in females, the reverse is true for isolated cleft palate where more girls than boys are affected.

Pathology

The term 'cleft palate' refers to a broad range of malformations affecting the hard or soft palate, usually occuring *in utero* and present at birth. However, some deformities, similar to these congenital defects, can come about later in life as a result of severe injury to the oral structure or to surgery which is usually associated with the treatment of malignant tumours.

A cleft of the lip involves the soft tissue extending through the vermilion border (the red part of upper lip) towards the nostril. The cleft may be incomplete, resulting in a minor notch, or complete, including all of the lip and up into the floor of the nostril. A cleft lip may be unilateral, involving one side, or bilateral, involving both sides. Cleft lip usually accompanies a cleft of the alveolus or dental arch which encircles the hard palate and supports the structures for the teeth. This may be slight, resulting in a notch in the alveolus, or extensive.

The anterior two-thirds of the palate is the hard palate which is made up of the maxillary and palatine bones of the skull. The soft palate or velum consists of approximately one third of the palate. This structure is composed of muscle and mucosa and moves superiorly and posteriorly in concert with the posterior and lateral pharyngeal walls to separate the nasal and oral-pharyngeal spaces during speech and swallowing. A cleft palate is a fissure in the palatal tissue. A complete cleft of the lip and palate extends from the lip, through the alveolar arch, and the hard and soft palates, including the uvula. Isolated cleft palate may present as a complete cleft of the hard and soft palate, the posterior one-third of the hard palate and the soft palate, or the soft palate only. A minor defect of the uvula is sometimes termed bifid uvula which, in itself, may well be asymptomatic. In submucous cleft palate, the palate appears to be structurally intact but there are bony and muscular defects under the mucosa that may be barely visible on the surface. The muscular deficit is the main cause of symptoms (Weatherley White *et al.*, 1972).

Whilst cleft lip and cleft palate are readily detected, clefts of the soft palate or submucous cleft palate may go undetected for some time, even into middle life despite disordered speech (Velasco *et al.*, 1988). A difficulty with feeding is one of the symptoms which should alert the physician to examine the palate in more detail. All those symptomatic patients in one cohort of patients with submucous cleft, examined by Moss, reported feeding difficulties from birth to 12 months. A high proportion of people with submucous clefts were found to have speech problems, with nasal escape and hypernasal resonance, and associated faults of articulation. Many had severe ear, nose and throat problems with chronic secretory otitis media (Moss *et al.*, 1988). However, these authors stressed that submucous cleft can be asymptomatic whereas cleft of the soft palate always results in speech difficulties.

Although there have been great advances in the operative treatment of cleft lip and palate, there is very poor information regarding the underlying, normal anatomy of the associated areas. Detailed studies of the palatopharyngeus, palatoglossus and the muscles of the uvula, are almost non-existent. There remain debates about the blood supply, and the innervation to these muscle groups, and thus details regarding the anatomical impairment of cleft palate are lacking. The function of the normal eustachian tube is not agreed upon and there are limited studies on tongue anatomy (Bluestone, 1971; Spriestersbach *et al.*, 1973).

Hearing Problems Associated with Cleft Palate and Submucous Cleft Palate

Middle-ear diseases such as secretory otitis media (SOM) and chronic otitis media, leading to hearing loss, occur very frequently among children with cleft palate with or without associated cleft lip (Grant, 1988).

In most studies the frequency of decreased hearing level was found to be between 50 and 100%, being more problematic before the closure of the palate (Fria, 1987). There are some abnormalities in the cleft palate population, which may predispose these children to middle-ear effusion. They include altered base of skull anatomy, abnormal positioning of the tensor and levator palati muscles and reflux of oropharyngeal secretions into the nasal pharynx (Gordon *et al.*, 1988). These authors conducted a retrospective study reviewing the incidence and nature of ear disease in 50 adolescent patients, who had cleft palates repaired in infancy. Half the patients had a history of grommet insertion which did not result in better long-term hearing but was strongly associated with tympanosclerosis. Despite this, surprisingly, the authors recommend that 'at the time of palatal repair, grommets should be inserted to improve hearing in these infants'.

Furthermore, a recent study of 44 eleven-year-old children, born with complete unilateral cleft lip and palate showed a high incidence of hearing impairment and abnormal middle ear pressure, but remarkably no association was found between the grommet insertion and hearing impairment. This study found a greater risk of associated problems with grommet insertion and recommended reservations about the indiscriminate use of grommets (Ovesen and Blegvad-Anderson, 1992). Despite these studies grommet insertion is, in practice, a very common procedure used with this population particularly during the early years as speech develops. The controversy was addressed by Robinson *et al.* (1992) in a multi-centre, prospective, controlled study of 110 consecutive cleft palate children. This concluded that ventilation tubes had no long-term effect on otitis media effusion, treated and untreated groups showing similar results. There was however, a significant difference in the mean hearing thresholds, with the treated group having better hearing. These authors suggested a compromise of unilateral insertion of a short-stay grommet.

Surgical Management of Patients with Cleft Lip and Palate

It is not the place of this review to conduct a detailed investigation of surgical procedures associated with the cleft lip, palate repair and velopharyngeal insufficiency. However, it is important to say that there is still very little evidence that assists with choosing one procedure above another and in determining the timing of operation in terms of gaining a better outcome. Whilst, in theory, many propose that different surgical techniques are more appropriate according to the type and breadth of the cleft, most of the information is anecdotal and descriptive and there have been few randomly controlled trials.

It is likely that different surgical techniques may have a different impact upon articulation, speech, resonance and hearing. However, it has been argued that certain surgeons become skilful at certain procedures and that it is this skill and not the procedure that is important to the final result.

Timing of Repair

One of the issues that has been debated long and hard is whether primary cleft palate surgery should be performed before the child is two years of age. There are concerns that early cleft palate surgery is harmful to the subsequent facial growth and development. Recently, a report by

Ross (1987) examined 1600 cephalometric radiographs from 16 treatment groups and evaluated the effects of different surgical timing on the development of the maxillofacial structures. He summarizes his findings as:

> The overall conclusion must be that there is not a great deal of difference in facial growth related to the age of hard and soft palate repair, but the data seemed to favour early repair in the first year of life as having a slight advantage over the medium and the late repair groups which were not as good.

Similarly the effect of age at primary palatal repair on speech was investigated in a group of 108 consecutive children whose palates were repaired between 12.9 months and 22.1 months. The results showed that the children who were operated on between the ages of 12 and 18 months developed significantly better speech than those operated on later. Three-quarters of the early group had normal speech as compared to less than a quarter of those operated on at around 22 months. Additionally, more children in the second group required further surgery to eliminate the signs of cleft palate speech associated with velopharyngeal inadequacy (Haapanen and Rantala, 1992).

Type of Repair

There are three main surgical procedures; the 'V-Y retroposition', the 'von Langenbeck' procedure and 'the delayed hard palate closure'. The results of palatal repair are commonly assessed, first by the status of speech and then by the adequacy of maxillofacial development. Frequently, in reports, the specific criteria for judging outcomes of both have been either vague, or widely differing.

A review of the results of two different surgical procedures, the von Langenbeck (simple closure) and the V-Y retroposition, for repair of the clefts of the soft palate only was undertaken by Musgrave, McWilliams and Matthews (1975). The authors were detailed in their analysis of associated speech dimensions including nasal resonance, articulation, and also hoarseness, which is very frequently overlooked. The two groups of children were compared and judged to be similar in intelligence, language and articulation at the time of surgery. The simple closure group was, at first, found to be slightly more hoarse than the V-Y repair group, while the latter was found to have slightly more hypernasality. Hearing acuity was somewhat poorer in the simple closure group and the need for secondary surgical procedures was noticeably greater in the simple closure group. The authors suggest that while the findings are not conclusive, they do add to the existing evidence that the V-Y repair probably yields a somewhat better initial speech result than the simple closure repair although the differences between groups were found to be small; speech adequacy was achieved in the V-Y retroposition group with less need for secondary surgery, which is a highly important and critical difference.

A study by Spauwen, Goorhuis-Brouwer and Schutte (1992) compared the Furlow cleft palate repair with the von Langenbeck. Twenty children were entered into this prospective study and randomly allocated into two groups. In both groups, a two-stage procedure was applied except in the cases of cleft of the soft palate only. The results suggested that the Furlow technique proved to be superior to the von Lagenbeck technique as far as speech quality was concerned: at the mean age of 3.5 years nasality and nasal escape were absent in 'almost all cases'. However, there was no significant difference between the techniques in respect of articulatory skills, language comprehension, language production and hearing. The authors note that the Furlow technique is more difficult to perform, particularly in wide clefts.

The Zurich approach offers a different management approach to patients with cleft lip and palate. The soft palate is repaired at approximately 18 months, the theory being that there is more tissue available for achieving 'adequate velar-links' at that age. The hard palate is repaired at the age of 5 years. Interestingly, one of the concerns regarding late repair of the hard palate has been related to the suggestions that before the operation children develop compensatory techniques which impede normal articulation after the operation. However, a study reported by Van Demark et al. (1989) found very acceptable speech articulation, voice quality and velopharyngeal competency of subjects with complete unilateral cleft lip and palate treated in one centre. Subjects were rated as exhibiting adequate to marginal velopharyngeal competency 94.5% of the time and the incidence of compensatory articulation errors was low. They suggest that this is probably related to the age at the time of the soft palate repair, which may contribute to the better speech outcome of the subjects. A further factor was the specialized nature of the small team involved in the management of this population. The unreplicated and surprising success of this series is noticeable when one compares it to a study reported by Wu, Chen and Noordhoff (1988), which investigated retrospectively a group of 47 Chinese children who had their soft palates repaired at 18 months and the hard palate closed at 6–7 years. There were a high number of compensatory articulatory errors, with particular difficulty with affricates, prior to the hard palate being repaired. As other studies have found, the articulation error types showed that sound substitution occurred more frequently followed by omission and distortion.

Thus, controversy is still reflected in the literature relating to the various approaches to palatal repair. In addition to the issues of surgical technique and the time of the surgery, there are other issues which have been raised but not satisfactorily answered. One of these issues is the size of the adenoids and the importance of this in speech results following primary palatoplasty. A study by Gereau and Shprintzen (1988), analysed the speech results relative to adenoid size of 100 normal children, 138 children with clefts associated with syndromes and 850 children with non-syndromic clefts. The data suggested a strong positive correlation between the incidence of hypernasal resonance postpalatoplasty and relative adenoid size in the cleft children. Velar-adenoidal closure, the use of the adenoid to obstruct the nasal airway when the velum was raised, was consistently observed in both cleft and normal children. These authors conclude that there is clear evidence that the adenoids play a crucial role in the development of normal speech. This again raises the interesting issue of the timing of palate repair. The adenoids would not be well developed until 12–18 months and surgery at 6 months might result in less efficient closure and a longer period for compensatory articulation to be learned (Musgrave *et al.*, 1975).

There has also been debate about the most effective treatment for submucous cleft palate. Some schools of thought suggest that any submucous cleft palate should be surgically repaired. Velasco *et al.* (1988), however, suggest that the decisions regarding surgery should be left until speech is developed. Theses authors reviewed the files of 180 patients with unrepaired submucous cleft palates and found velopharyngeal insufficiency was present in only 53% of the cases. The authors speculated that these may have been due to a specific malformation of the musculus uvulae in certain types of submucous cleft. The combination of unrepaired submucous cleft, and velopharyngeal insufficiency, due to malformation of the muculus uvulae seemed to lead to a significantly higher incidence of conductive hearing loss which may, again, be related to the relationship between the velar muscle malformation and the eustachian tube malfunction. The possible abnormalities of the musculus uvulae can be detected by the use of video nasendoscopy and videofluoroscopy (Albery *et al.*, 1986).

Clinical experience from primary palatoplasty and studies of velopharyngeal valving suggests that the intravelar veloplasty (IVVP) could increase the achievement of velopharyngeal competence in patients undergoing pharyngeal flap surgery. This hypothesis was tested by Jarvis and Trier (1988), comparing retrospectively 91 patients who had undergone superiorly based pharyngeal flap surgery with intravelar veloplasty with 39 patients who underwent the same procedure but without the veloplasty. Although the theory seems sound that the IVVP would improve pharyngeal competence, there was no difference between these two groups, over 92% of both groups achieving adequacy by objective measures. It is possible that IVVP, when added to the pharyngeal flap operation has no particular effect as the flap operation already produces competence. Methods of detecting patients who require the additional intervention need to be developed.

Another retrospective study, Hall *et al.*, 1991, reviewing patients with a history of cleft palate, who had pharyngeal flap surgery as adults, demonstrated that when the surgery is undertaken at this later age, the outcome of speech is less good and tends to be related to the pre-operative articulation. This study would suggest that the response to speech therapy, prior to surgery, may predict the outcome of surgery. Of the patients reported in the study, 10 were referred for intensive speech therapy pre- and postoperatively and whilst there is very little detail in this paper about the nature of therapy, it was noted that half of the patients who were non-compliant had postoperative intelligibility which was not markedly better than their pre-operative speech and this was different from those who complied with treatment whose post-operative speech was better. There are indications from this study that early surgical intervention to correct velopalatal incompetence, along with speech therapy to prevent compensatory articulation, would more likely have better, long-term results.

Most of the studies reported here show methodological and other deficiencies which in many cases cast doubts over their conclusions. Sell (1994, personal communication) draws attention to the extensive descriptions of surgery in this literature compared with the cursory information on outcomes. A review by Sell (in preparation) outlines some of the inadequacies including: (a) inadequacies of speech assessments, e.g. use of undefined terms such as 'average speech', 'intelligible speech'; (b) selection of one speech characteristic, e.g. nasal escape; (c) no data or listener reliability; (d) the use of biased observers; and (e) small sample sizes.

In order to overcome some of these difficulties in comparing outcomes Dalston et al. (1988), proposed a set of minimum standards for reporting the results of surgery in this specialized area, detailing procedures for ensuring reliable and valid judgements concerning anatomic integrity, aesthetics, functional integrity and speech assessments. The standards suggest conformity so that comparisons can be made. This paper should assist all members of the cleft palate team to share a common approach in furthering the knowledge in this area and to group and compare clinical data more easily.

Nature of a Speech Disorder Related to Cleft Palate and Velopharyngeal Insufficiency

Introduction

The majority of persons with treated palatal clefts have no serious problems with speech or communication. However, approximately 25% of them fail to develop adequate speech (Spriestersbach et al. 1973). There is evidence that the presence of long-standing speech problems is related to management early in life. It is possible that different surgical and speech therapy approaches and cultural differences, may lead to different levels and types of speech difficulty. It is too easy to assume that the speech/language difficulties are entirely related to the persistent structural problems involving palatal function, malocclusion, hearing difficulties, and fistulae, etc. Many studies suggest more complex attributions such as, more limited opportunity to swallow, suck and speak, resulting in less developed oral motor/oral and sensory systems, different child/parent interaction and less opportunity to interact positively in infant play. In general, persons with cleft palate are at risk of disorders of articulation, resonance, voice; and reduced intelligibility, phonology and language.

Underlying causes of speech disorders

Craniofacial anomalies affect the oral and vocal tract and can influence the health of the hearing mechanisms. Thus, the process of normal speech and language development is compromised in fundamental ways. The pre-speech neurological patterning of movements of the tongue, lips and the velopharyngeal valve, which might take place *in utero* and after birth, may be affected by the structural abnormalities. It is probable that the sensory motor pre-speech movements of the oral and pharyngeal musculature, which are developed through fetal sucking, may not develop normally and could contribute to problems in feeding and perhaps speech development later.

Theories regarding the aerodynamic regulation of the larynx on airflow into the oral space have been discussed as a possible cause of speech difficulties. If a person wishes to reduce the amount of hypernasality and nasal emission then a reduced amount of airflow is one compensatory technique. However this compensation may put the larynx under some stress.

Adequate intraoral pressure is important for the normal production of consonants. Warren, Dalston and Dalston (1990), investigated the factors that differentiated cleft palate speakers who achieve adequate oral pressures from those who did not. The most important significant factor differentiating these two groups was found to be the magnitude of nasal plus velopharyngeal resistance, which in turn relates to the compensatory articulation which may be developed to control air-flow and to develop the necessary intraoral pressures.

It would seem to follow that patients with bilateral collapse of the primary and secondary palate might well have more difficulty in compressing air for the production of some consonants. A retrospective study of 166 subjects by Dalston, Warren and Dalston (1992), concluded that patients with bi-lateral complete cleft were more likely than patients with uni-lateral complete cleft, or palate only cleft, to manifest compensatory articulation that might be related to the inability to produce correct air pressure. Patients who manifested compensatory articulation were more likely to have larger nasal cross-sectional errors than those without compensatory articulation.

These findings, if they are supported, suggest that children with large nasal airways may be at increased risk of developing abnormal speech patterns, which will be harder to overcome with therapy. Such children may well be candidates for relatively early palate repair.

Disorders of voice resonance and consonant articulation are the usual problems found in the group who persist in having difficulties despite primary procedures designed to provide intact and functional oral structures (Wells, 1971). Whilst the articulation and phonological problems are well documented, there is less detailed description related to associated vocal disturbance problems, such as hoarseness, breathlessness, reduced loudness or abnormal pitch with restricted pitch range, which have been observed being of higher incidence in individuals with cleft palate. Zajac and Linville (1989) and D'Antonio *et al.* (1988) report that 41% of a group of individuals with velopharyngeal insufficiency exhibited abnormal vocal quality.

Palatal surgery is almost bound to improve vocalization and resonance. The phonetic deviance may be improved but it is unclear whether the underlying disturbance to the oropharyngeal area is influenced rapidly. O'Gara and Logemann (1985) report a predominance of glottal articulations in pre-linguistic vocalizations of cleft palate children. Comparisons of vocalizations pre- and post-operatively, demonstrated that these children rapidly recovered from the surgery to assume a pattern of speech that demonstrated a whole range of articulatory placements in use and similarities in the phonotactic structures with those of normal children. The main difference, when comparing the speech of cleft palate children, both pre- and post-operatively, with that of normal children is the marked lack of front (i.e. bi-labial and apical oblique line laminal) contoids with a high predominance of glottal and velar sounds (Grunwell and Russell 1987; O'Gara and Logemann 1985).

The degree of velopharyngeal insufficiency may be predicted to some extent on the perceptual assessment. The presence of nasal turbulence suggested a smaller velopharyngeal gap, despite the severe distortion of speech.

A comparison of velopharyngeal gap size in patients with hypernasality concluded that it is possible to detect the gap size and concluded that those who had nasal rustle as a primary speech characteristic should consider speech therapy prior to surgery as it may well be amenable to change conservatively, whereas those who have hypernasal emission and hypernasality without turbulence may well not benefit from speech therapy without surgical intervention (Kummer *et al.*, 1992). This study analysed the differences between 10 patients with hypernasality and audible nasal emission and 10 patients with nasal turbulence. They did not go on to confirm their suggestions regarding therapy timing.

It is suggested that these organic predispositions to speech difficulty may be added to by psychological stresses. The traumatic effect of giving birth to an impaired baby can, in itself, result in negative interaction between the mother and child and problems with bonding (Witzell, 1990). An analysis of discourse between a parent and a cleft palate child and a non-cleft palate sibling demonstrated the parent's interaction with the cleft palate child were less successful and more negative and it was more difficult for a topic of conversation to be maintained than with the non-cleft palate child (Lynch *et al.*, 1988).

Chapman (1991) compared five toddlers with cleft lip and palate and five non-cleft toddlers aged 12–14 months. Spontaneous vocalizations demonstrated a clear difference between the frequency and type of consonant productions. The toddlers with cleft lip and palate produced markedly fewer vocalizations and even taking this into account, fewer consonants overall. There were also qualitative differences in the consonant inventories, with fewer stop consonants used by cleft palate children.

There appear to be some similarities in the error types of very young cleft palate children. Powers, Dunn and Erickson (1990) in a study of four children between the ages of 3 and 4 years with surgically repaired clefts, demonstrated that there are marked similarities in errors with regard to their phonetic inventories. The frequency and type of phonological process differed however. These differences could be related to the different levels of language ability. The authors again stress that the articulatory problems among children may not only be a result of the structural deficit and that there may well be a complex group of underlying predisposing factors.

Maternal interactive behaviour is affected by the needs of the child. A study of children with speech related anomalies compared with non-speech related anomalies and controls indicated very specific adaptations on the part of the mother in compensation (Wasserman *et al.*, 1988). The mothers of children with speech related anomalies were more likely to take charge of the flow of their free play interactions, tended to initiate and make use of specific techniques that controlled and paced the focus of the child's attention. This study shows that maternal interactive behaviour did not seem to be global but specific, in response to the child's difficulties.

There is strong evidence that there are severe psychosocial difficulties associated with oral facial defects. Problems with self concept, social perception by peers, parents, teachers and the public may lead to difficulties in self-confidence and conduct problems at home and at school. In a review of 104 patients with oral facial defects, Broder and Strauss (1991) found that 56% of patients exhibited problems that would warrant a psychosocial referral. Males with clefts were more apt to have behaviour problems, lower achievement and unresolved family difficulties. The review supported the notion that increasing age seemed to be associated with increased psychosocial difficulties. Intelligibility and diagnostic category of the speech disorder and facial disfigurement were significantly associated with the patient's psychosocial status.

The same authors studied 102 patients with cleft lip, cleft palate or both from ages of 13–19 years to investigate their views with regard to appearance, speech ability and intelligibility. There was concordance in the ratings between parents and children and whilst more than half were very satisfied with their appearance, articulation intelligibility and speech ability, a high proportion expressed concern in all three issues. Again, these issues do not seem to resolve with age and may well need to be acknowledged as requiring attention in the rehabilitation process (Strauss *et al.*, 1988).

Assessment of Palatal Function

Considerable research has been conducted in an attempt to develop valid and reliable measures of velopharyngeal function. Some of these are based on instrumental techniques and others depend on specialist assessment by experienced listeners who rate the articulation, nasality, nasal emission and vocal tone of the patient. The most commonly employed tools used to evaluate velopharyngeal function include nasendoscopy and videofluoroscopy and nasal anemometry and nasometry. The latter two of these are not invasive and are used frequently to assist speech and language therapists in their listener judgement.

Hypernasality is a parameter of cleft palate speech that has elicited a huge amount of research. An important goal in rehabilitation is the elimination or reduction of hypernasality and thus it is important that objective, reliable, valid and comparable methods are used. Listener judgements have been used commonly but, because of the poor reliability of individual listener judgements, group judgements are favoured in research (McWillaims *et al.*, 1981).

Instrumental methods offer objective, but indirect, information on hypernasality. However, the instrumental measurements must also be subjectively interpreted in relation to perception, as a problem with hypernasality is only a problem if it is perceived as such by listeners (Bzoch, 1989).

Phonetic content has been shown to influence the perception of whether cleft palate speech is defective or not, thus contributing to the perception of inconsistency of cleft palate speech defects and to the difficulty of evaluating speech parameters such as hypernasality. For example, some vowels are judged to be more frequently hypernasal than others. Bzoch maintains that hypernasality can only be truly and reliably evaluated in the absence of articulation disorders and when phonation is clear. Bzoch advocates a test using words which are said alternately with the nares being occluded (e.g. by pinching the nose) and opened. A change in clarity between the two would indicate some degree of hypernasality. Haapanen developed this approach further resulting in a simple and more reliable measure of assessing the degree of hypernasality (Haapanen, 1991).

Hardin *et al.* (1992) investigated the relationship between nasalance scores assessed by nasometry and perceptual judgements of nasality, for 74 subjects, 51 with cleft palate and 23 non-cleft controls. Twenty-nine of the 51 subjects with cleft palate had received pharyngeal flap surgery. The sensitivity, specificity and efficiency of the nasometer as a screening instrument was analysed. There was 91% agreement of the classification based on nasometry. However, the results were less good for subjects who had had pharyngeal flaps. The authors of this study concur with others that perceiving hypernasality (which may be more evident in patients with pharyngeal flaps) is difficult and requires more experienced listeners; this may be one of the reasons why this study demonstrates some degree of disparity in the findings.

This discrepancy between experienced and less experienced listeners is even more clearly differentiated when one compares speech ratings by speech clinicians and those done by parents and children. Ratings of speech samples of children with cleft palate were obtained from speech clinicians in cleft palate clinic, speech clinicians in schools, parents of children with clefts, parents of children without clefts, and children with and without clefts (Starr *et al.*, 1984). Analyses of the obtained ratings, which were acknowledgedly rather gross, showed that speech clinicians, parents and children with hypernasal speech rate similarly. Both groups of speech clinicians findings correlated more closely than other groups. In addition, the speech clinicians seemed to be more discerning regarding articulation ratings than the other groups. In general, speech clinicians' judgements of nasality were representative of other listener groups. However, their ratings of articulation seem to be different, perceiving a wider range of difficulties.

According to Dalston, Warren and Dalston (1991a,b), nasalance scores obtained from the nasometer correspond well with clinical judgements of hypernasilty and hyponasality. However, in this study the clinical impressions of resonance were obtained from a single trained listener. A follow-up study by Nellis, Neiman and Lehman (1992) was conducted using ten trained listeners. This study showed that the judges had more difficulty in detecting hyponasality than hypernasality and the ratings by the judges differed as a result of the phonetic context affecting their perception, as the perceptual characteristics and phonetic variation can mask or enhance the acoustic realisation of nasality differences. One could conclude that the use of a nasometer along with experienced listening, can assist with getting more reliable results. Thus, any study of outcome may be affected, not only by the listeners skill but also by the tasks that the patient is asked to do. Dalston and Seaver (1992) demonstrated this in a comparison of rating two reading passages, the Zoo Passage and the Rainbow Passage with nasometry and listener judgements. The latter passage showed less correspondence between judgements of nasality, and nasometry (and other judgements), whereas the Zoo Passage tended to give a better relationship. It was felt that the Rainbow Passage is syntactically more complex giving patients more overall difficulty. The striking point to learn from this piece of work is that the material used in the assessment can, itself, affect the perceived outcome.

It has been speculated that measuring intraoral pressure would assist with gauging the velopharyngeal adequacy. However, this is being found to be only partially true. In a study by Dalston et al. (1988) the intraoral pressure was measured on 267 patients, articulating the word 'hamper'. The results indicated that for patients with small deviations, pressure reduced as the extent of velopharyngeal impairment increased. However, most of the patients with larger velopharyngeal impairments were able to produce an intraoral pressure of 30 mm. H_2O, even when the impairment was such that intraoral and intranasal pressures were, essentially, equal. Obviously these subjects had learned to maintain an intraoral pressure despite their velopharyngeal impairment. This may have been by blocking with their tongue, or other articulatory compensatory moves. Thus, the use of intraoral pressure is useful only to a limited extent.

These compensatory behaviours do make it difficult to assess cleft palate speech in an objective way. Some clients have compensatory behaviours that impede their normal speech production. Others have compensatory behaviours which are poorly developed or which facilitate speech improvement. Comparison of the intraoral pressure of 74 subjects with cleft palate with that of a control group of 137 subjects with adequate velopharyngeal closure, showed that a loss of resistance of the velo-port was compensated by an increase in resistance at the nasal port. Airflow rate appears to be adjusted to total upper airway resistance. These findings support the hypothesis by the authors that the speech system is constrained to meet aero-dynamic requirements (Laine et al., 1988).

Speech and Language Therapy – Description

Treatment of communication disorders

Cleft palate can predispose the person to language, phonation, resonance and phonological disorders. Whereas the language disorder is similar to that of other children and would be treated in the same way, the phonatory resonance and phonological disorders are different and will be dealt with in this section.

Treatment of disorders of phonation

Some patients with cleft palate will have hyperfunctional voice, some hypofunctional voice, and some will have vocal cord nodules associated with aberrant phonation. As with any other therapy, it is important that the assessment should indicate the cause of the disorder to assist with targeting the therapy appropriately. If the phonation problem is associated with velopharyngeal incompetence and an effort on the part of the patient to reduce nasal emission by valving with the vocal cords, the treatment is associated with removing the underlying cause, i.e. the velopharyngeal insufficiency.

Some children may develop a voice disorder as they grow older and their valving mechanism becomes less efficient with growth. Thus, it is important that phonation is monitored along with the other aspects of speech and language at the regular follow-ups. Most of the recommended methods of improving phonation with the cleft palate person are similar to those with voice disorders not associated with clefts. Behaviour modification techniques using rewards or more appropriate use of the voice are particularly useful for young children who tend to vocally abuse (Boone and McFarlane, 1988).

Many children who have had fluctuating hearing problems related to their cleft palate may have become accustomed to using their voice at an incorrect volume. It is generally recommended that direct teaching methods to assist the child in identifying appropriate volume can be of assistance. All authors describing this form of therapy stress the importance of self-monitoring.

The usual techniques of respiration and relaxation are employed with this client group, as with other client groups with voice disorders. When vocal cord nodules are present, the aim is to reduce hyperfunction. But it must be remembered that these phonation disorders are compensatory behaviours and changing the compensatory behaviour may affect the primary problem, leading to increased hypernasality and nasal emission. Frequently voice therapy can only be undertaken as part of the overall management of the disorder.

> 'We know of no research that has been carried out to assess the results of therapy in children or adults with the phonation problems sometimes secondary to aberrant velopharyngeal valve' (McWilliams et al., 1990).

Treatment of disorders of resonance

Speech and language therapy procedures to reduce or eliminate hypernasality were described many decades ago (Young, 1928). Despite this, there is little evidence that speech and language therapy to reduce hypernasality does modify the problem. Therapy is based on the underlying assumption that if hypernasality is modified, then the velopharyngeal closure will be improved. However, this does not necessarily follow. It is generally considered unlikely that speech and language therapy can do anything to improve hypernasality if the mechanism is substantially inadequate. Most experienced clinicians now suggest that speech and language therapy should wait for several months after surgical intervention, as patients may spontaneously improve their speech without direct intervention. However, if direct intervention is required, a number of traditional techniques may assist. Boone and McFarlane (1988), suggest eight therapeutic approaches for treating hypernasality.

1. Experimenting with increased loudness.
2. Ear training to assist with discrimination between oral and nasal resonance.
3. Evaluating the effects of lowering the speaker's pitch.
4. Explaining the nature of the problem so that the speaker understands clearly what is to be modified.
5. Providing as much auditory and kinaesthetic feedback as possible from nasal and oral resonance.
6. Developing increased oral opening in cases where the oral port is restricted.
7. Assessing the positive or negative effects of placing the voice by focusing on the facial mask.
8. Training respiration to increase loudness.

Discriminant training has been stressed for many years (Fisher, 1975). This is said to be particularly useful for patients who are able to produce normal resonance for individual or short passages of speech, but whose speech deteriorates in conversation. In this technique the patient learns to discriminate between the target and the deviant pattern. Then a programme to develop self-monitoring is planned, with the patient being actively involved in rating their own speech efforts.

Reducing oral breath pressure on fricatives and stop consonants has been thought to reduce perceived hypernasality, but again relies on good self-monitoring. Self-monitoring can be improved by the patient alternating purposefully between normal and hypernasal speech. Learning the ability to swop between these three forms of resonance can assist them to control their own production (McWilliams, 1981). No research evidence has been found to indicate which of these techniques is more favourable or more efficacious.

Bio-feedback Methods

Early therapy often includes the use of simple visual feedback to give information. The use of a mirror or candle can demonstrate to the speaker the degree of nasal escape. The goal is to learn to eliminate inappropriate airflow by closing the velopharyngeal sphincter. More sophisticated bio-feedback methods have been described since the 1970s but few of these have been properly evaluated. However, Fletcher (1978) attested his highly specific programme using TONAR, which gives a reinforcement display in both analogue and digital form. The speech pathologists can manipulate the goal-ratio dial on the instrument panel so that an actual utterance can be compared with the stated goal. The success counter permits easy record keeping and speakers are kept constantly informed of their success. Fletcher tested this programme on 19 children with hypernasality and a nasalance level averaging 40%. The programme was individual and intensive and each child participated in 13 sessions over a period of a week, with each session lasting 20–30 mins. Fletcher found great variability in the nasalance modification. Eight of the 19 subjects met the 85% success criteria of 15% or less nasalance on at least two sub-sets of sentences and were able to maintain that level. Five were successful on one or more sub-sets but could not maintain the performance. Five showed some reduction in nasalance but were highly erratic and maintenance was very poor. One subject did not modify the nasalance percentage and surgical or prosthetic intervention was recommended. The evidence from this study is difficult to interpret as many of the subjects may well have had inadequate velopharyngeal mechanisms. Additionally, this approach to therapy was not compared with a different approach so it is difficult to interpret whether the subjects improved because of the feedback system itself, or because of other factors such as the intensity of exposure to therapy. It would appear that this systematic approach might be successful with individuals who can achieve velopharyngeal closure but who do this inconsistently.

In a review of therapy for hypernasality, McWilliams (1981) concluded that speech therapy for improving hypernasality does not appear to be warranted in many cases:

> It may be helpful for those borderline speakers for whom surgical treatment or prosthetics is either unwarranted or unwanted, for those patients who have had pharyngeal flaps or those for whom appliances have been made and who need to learn efficient use of the new mechanism.

The specialist therapists caution that the use of therapy to reduce hypernasality, where the mechanism is inadequate, could be destructive and may well result in voice disturbances and complicate other communication difficulties. When discussing treatment of these disorders and their likelihood of success, Skolnick and McCall (1973) advised clinicians to 'think Sphincter' and undertake therapy only when valve competence or potential for competence can be demonstrated.

Treatment of articulatory and phonological disorders

Traditional articulation therapy is usually considered appropriate for speech problems associated with cleft palate. In most cases these speech problems are clearly viewed as articulation disorders, resulting from a structural defect or inadequacy or associated learned compensatory technique. The treatment strategy adopted is designed to achieve 'the correct production of deviant consonant sounds in isolation, syllables, single words, sentences and finally, in everyday speech' (Albery and Enderby, 1984).

Difficulties in achieving these aims are frequently reported, most often in regard to generalizing to everyday speech. Most authors (Hahn, 1989; Phillips, 1979; Smith, 1969) stressed the importance of developing articulation along with vocabulary and interactive general communication.

Morley (1970) listed four goals of speech therapy for persons with clefts:

1. Teaching oral direction of the breath stream for the purpose of learning to use the palatal and pharyngeal muscles to control the velopharyngeal sphincter.
2. Coordinating the neuro-muscular control of the velopharyngeal muscles with other articulatory muscles.
3. Teaching correct articulation of all consonants and vowels and the ability to use those sounds in all positions in words and in blends as well.
4. Introducing the newly learned sounds into speech establishing the unconscious use of new and correct habits of articulation.

Morley organized articulation training according to principles of motor learning, which involves inhibition of faulty articulation patterns already developed, facilitating required movements, association of the new movements with auditory kinaesthetic and touch-pressure feedback, and stabilization of the new performance at an automatic level. Whilst many of Morley's suggestions are still seen as salient, her recommendations on appropriate age to treat has been challenged. She felt that it was not appropriate to do very much for the children under 4 years of age except to attempt to teach oral direction of the air-stream. Morley was an early advocate of group therapy and also was in advance of her time in promoting the necessity to avoid tension associated with glottal and pharyngeal substitutions. She detailed the steps required in therapy and always took into account the limitations imposed by any existing velopharyngeal incompetence (Morley, 1970).

Grunwell and Dive (1988) suggest that, along with an articulation disorder, cleft palate children frequently have a phonological problem. This study is one of the few that have evaluated a therapy approach. Even this, however, is limited, having reported the progress of only two children. The children received an intensive therapy course of both articulatory and phonological therapy. Detailed articulation and phonological assessments after therapy demonstrated a 're-organizational expansion of previously static phonological systems, sometimes in spite of persisting articulatory disabilities and sometimes accompanied by improvements in the articulatory abilities'. The results of the study were interpreted by the authors as demonstrating that speech development can become arrested at a certain stage in phonological acquisition as a result of articulatory disability.

Empirical evidence regarding the effectiveness of articulation therapy for patients with cleft palate is limited in both its quantity and design. Experimental control is often difficult and the subjects are bound to be heterogenous with different types of cleft, surgical interventions, hearing abilities, language backgrounds, intelligence, education, age, etc. Additionally, descriptions of therapy are frequently not detailed enough and the programmes tend to have limited goals, which do not permit definitive statements about the value of complex treatments delivered to patients over prolonged periods.

Prins and Bloomer (1965) evaluated the effectiveness of an 8 week intensive residential speech programme for 10 children with reported cleft palates, which combined both group and individual treatment. The children improved their scores on word intelligibility, but there was little direct evidence that the therapy programme resolved conversational speech.

Chisum et al.(1969) evaluated articulation therapy delivered to children who had either hypernasal speech, speech with nasal emission or a combination of both. All the children were thought to have borderline velopharyngeal competence. The subjects ranged between 6 and 12 years and received half-hour therapy sessions twice each week. Each subject was seen, individually, over an average period of 7 months and was taught to produce sounds in isolation and then in nonsense syllables, words, sentences and conversations. There was a significant difference between the experimental subjects and those in the control group, with gains made primarily on fricatives, which were the sounds stressed in the training programme. However, many of the subjects were left with some degree of articulation problem.

Harrison (1969) evaluated a language and speech stimulation programme for pre-school children with cleft palate. The approach was to develop the correct articulatory placements and to improve nasal emission and resonance. Articulation tests before and after treatment demonstrated that both the experimental and control groups made gains but the experimental group made significantly greater gains.

Schendel and Bzoch (1970) evaluated an intensive summer residential speech therapy programme. Although no experimental control features were employed, the authors used a case study format to describe the gains made. The treatment programme was intended to provide an atmosphere 'conducive to learning'. If one makes the assumption that the speech of the children would have been stable without therapy at the time of the programme, then the evidence presented is favourable to articulation therapy for cleft palate children. The lack of control makes it impossible to conclude that any particular treatment procedure used was especially effective. The data in this study indicated that children reduced the number of sounds mis-articulated on an articulation test and that the articulation errors that did persist were reduced in severity. This was true, even for the children who had remaining velopharyngeal incompetence.

Van Demark (1974) described two groups of Danish children between the ages of 5 and 7 years old. Subjects were classified as to whether they had evidence of velopharyngeal closure, marginal closure or velopharyngeal incompetence and assigned into two groups, one group receiving unspecified speech therapy and the other group receiving no treatment. In the group receiving speech therapy, all types of articulation errors, especially sound omissions, were decreased. The subjects who were judged to have good velopharyngeal closure made greater gains than those with marginal or incompetent closure. Of the children with marginal closure, those who received speech therapy made articulation gains, whereas children not in therapy did not. This study demonstrates that a group of children with cleft palate improved their articulation during a period in which speech therapy was provided. However, the study does indicate that not all speech problems related to velopharyngeal incompetence can be eliminated through speech therapy.

Shelton and Ruscello (1979) give descriptive information regarding the responses of patients with cleft palate or velopharyngeal insufficiency to articulation training, to bio-feedback intended to influence velopharyngeal function, or to the combination of these two procedures. Unfortunately there was no experimental control. Articulation training involved placement procedures, imitation practice, and reinforcement of correct responses. Subjects with presumed borderline velopharyngeal incompetence, as evidenced by nasal airflow during some but not all pressure consonants, made articulation gains with training. This study gives descriptions of individual patients and does demonstrate some interesting improvements, but the lack of a good way of classifying velopharyngeal insufficiency and the method of reporting the results makes it difficult to generalize the results.

Albery and Enderby (1984) compared the effectiveness of speech therapy delivered on two schedules, an intensive 6 week course and weekly therapy. The children had a mean age of 8.7 years and were assigned to two groups by random allocation. The children in the intensive group resided in the hospital during the weeks for the therapy period and the comparison group lived at home and received therapy from their local therapist. All subjects had velopharyngeal competence or near-competence as evidenced by freedom from hypernasality and little or no nasal escape as measured by nasal anemometry; most had repaired cleft palate or submucous cleft palate but a few had corrected pharyngeal disproportion or palatal incoordination. Children in intensive therapy were taught consonants in isolation, syllables, words, sentences and everyday speech. The two groups were assessed 1 month before treatment, immediately before treatment, at the end of treatment and at 6 monthly intervals after treatment through a 2 year post-treatment period. The pre-treatment data showed comparability between the groups. Following treatment the group receiving the intensive treatment were superior in their results on the articulation tests used. The gains were maintained and the intensive treatment group maintained its advantage relative to the comparison group over the 2 year period. Parents reported that children in the intensive group 'blossomed' becoming more competent and more verbal.

A study to determine the effectiveness of a 6 week intensive articulation therapy programme for 13 children with cleft palate or cleft lip and palate, and to investigate the maintenance of improvement of these children, was undertaken by Van Demark and Hardin (1986). This study was originally planned to have matched controls, but unfortunately, this was found to be 'impossible'. The subjects were considered to present velopharyngeal competence or marginal competence. Four hours of articulation therapy was given daily for 26 days. The speech progress was assessed immediately following the intensive therapy programme and again on a 9 month follow-up and these assessments were compared with the pre-treatment results. This study indicated that the subjects significantly improved their articulation performance during the programme but their progress was slower than had been expected. There was no significant difference between the articulation scores obtained immediately post therapy and those obtained during the 9 month follow-up examination, during which some subjects had received further therapy.

Some individual case studies have been discussed reporting progress with articulation therapy. One of note is Kawano *et al.* (1985) who described the response of speech therapy for an individual cleft palate girl, who substituted a laryngeal fricative for /S/ and /ʃ/. This detailed programme demonstrated the progress to more acceptable and desirable speech. Another single case study, using instrumental bio-feedback therapy for correction of articulation, is described by Michi *et al.* (1986). These authors employed a dynamic palatography in the successful correction of a Japanese 6-year-old girl with a repaired unilateral cleft and oral-nasal fistula. The therapy programme successfully reduced palatalization of many sounds. The child had 49 hourly sessions over a period of 1 year and maintained a substantial articulatory improvement, including the elimination of the tongue backing and air-stream lateralization. It was speculated by these authors that neither of those articulations would be likely to self-correct without structured therapy.

Conclusion

The literature relating to the efficacy of speech and language therapy in the treatment of cleft palate and velopharyngeal insufficiency is somewhat sparse. There are problems not only with regard to the quantity of research in the area but also quality of this research. There are substantial methodological problems in this very heterogenous group and there are debates regarding the reliability of different forms of assessment and the relationships of the different speech and language disorders. Despite this, the evidence in the literature would tentatively indicate that speech and language therapy for cleft palate children who have velopharyngeal competence or borderline competence is effective. It would appear that intensive, structured and targeted treatment has merit. However, the value of different approaches to treatment have not been compared.

There are many questions remaining to be answered. There has been little investigation of the effectiveness of surgery for cleft palate which have used convincing detailed specific speech and language tests as outcome measures. Many of the studies cited in our review have used rather gross measures which may not be sensitive to some of the specific aspects related to the quality of outcome of surgery.

Studies analysing the speech language and related pathology are robust and should act as a strong platform for further detailed enquiry relating to the nature, timing and delivery of therapy. Furthermore, whilst many speech and language therapists work with the parents of infants with cleft palate, to encourage good feeding and speech and language development, we have not found any studies which have evaluated the effectiveness of this preventative role. There are suggestions in the literature that feeding, swallowing and speech difficulties are related but there have been no studies that truly investigated this or whether modified feeding at an early age has an effect upon later speech and language development.

References

Albery E and Enderby P (1984). Intensive speech therapy for cleft palate children. British Journal of Disorders of Communication 19: 115–124.

Albery EH, Hathorn IS and Pigott RW (Eds) (1986). Cleft Lip and Palate: A Team Approach. Bristol: Wright.

Bluestone CD (1971). Eustachian tube obstruction in the infant with cleft palate. Annals of Otology Rhinology and Laryngology Suppl 2: 80.

Boone DR and McFarlane K (1988). The Voice and Voice Therapy. (4th Edition), Englewood Cliffs, NJ: Prentice-Hall.

Broder H and Strauss R (1991). Psychosocial problems and referrals among oral facial team patients. Journal of Rehabilitation Jan-Mar., 31–36.

Bzoch KR (1989). Measurement and assessment of categorical aspects of cleft palate speech. In: Bzoch KR (Ed) Communicative Disorders Related to Cleft Lip and Palate, 137–173. Boston: Little, Brown.

Chapman KL (1991). Vocalizations of toddlers with cleft lip and palate. Cleft Palate-Craniofacial Journal. 28(2): 172–178.

Chisum L, Shelton RL, Andt WB and Elbert M (1969). The relationship between remedial speech instruction activities and articulation change. Cleft Palate Journal 6: 57.

D'Antonio L, Muntz H, Province M and Marsh J. (1988). Laryngeal oblique line voice findings in patients with velopharyngeal disfunction. Laryngoscope 98: 432–438.

Dalston RM and Seaver EJ (1992). Relative values of various standardised passages in the nasometric assessments of patients with velopharyngeal impairments. Cleft Palate-Craniofacial Journal 29(1): 17–25.

Dalston RM, Warren DW and Dalston ET (1991a). The use of nasometry as a diagnostic tool for identifying patients with velopharyngeal impairment. Cleft Palate-Craniofacial Journal 28: 184–188.

Dalston RM, Warren DW and Dalston ET (1991b). The identification of nasal obstruction through clinical judgement of hyponasality and nasometric assessment of speech acoustics. American Journal of Orthodontics, Dentofac Orthop 100: 59–65.

Dalston RM, Warren DW and Dalston ET (1992). A preliminary study of nasal airway patency and its potential effect on speech performance. Cleft Palate-Craniofacial Journal 29(4): 330–335.

Dalston RM, Warren DW, Morr KE and Smith LR (1988). Intraoral pressure and its relationship to velopharyngeal inadequacy. Cleft Palate Journal 25(3): 210–219.

Dalston RM, Marsh J, Vig KW, Witzell MA and Bumsted RM (1988). Minimal standards for reporting the results of surgery on patients with cleft lip, cleft palate, or both: A proposal. Cleft Palate Journal 25(1): 3–7.

Fisher (1975). Improving Voice and Articulation. Houghton, Boston MA: Mifflin.

Fletcher SG (1978). Diagnosing Speech Disorders from Cleft Palate. New York: Grune and Stratton.

Fraser FC (1970). The genetics of cleft lip and palate. American Journal of Human Genetics 22: 336–352.

Fria TJ (1987). Conductive hearing loss in infants and young children with cleft palate. Journal of Paediatrics 111: 84–87.

Gereau SA and Shprintzen RJ (1988). The role of adenoids in the development of normal speech following palate repair. Laryngoscope 98: 299–303.

Gordon ASD, Jean-Louis F and Morton RP (1988). Late ear sequelae in cleft palate patients. International Journal of Pediatric Otorhinolaryngology 15: 149–156.

Gorlin RJ, Pindborg JJ and Cohen MM (1976). Syndromes of the Head and Neck. New York: McGraw-Hill.

Grant HR (1988). Cleft palate and glue ear. Archives of Diseases in Childhood 163: 176–179.

Grunwell P and Dive D (1988). Treating 'Cleft Palate Speech': Combining phonological techniques with traditional articulation therapy. Child Language Teaching and Therapy 4(2): 193–211.

Grunwell P and Russell J (1987). Vocalisations before and after cleft palate surgery: a pilot study. British Journal of Disorders of Communication 22: 1–17.

Haapanen ML (1991). A simple clinical method of evaluating perceived hypernasality. Folia Phoniatrica 43: 122–132.

Haapanen ML and Rantala SL (1992). Correlation between the age at repair and speech outcome in patients with isolated cleft palate. Scandinavian Journal of Plastic Reconstructive and Hand Surgery 26(1): 71–78.

Hahn E (1989). Directed home language stimulation programme for infants with cleft lip and palate. In: Bzoch KR (Ed) Communicative Disorders Related to Cleft Lip and Palate, (3rd Edition), 137. Boston, MA: Little, Brown.

Hall CD, Golding-Kushner KJ, Argamaso RV and Strauch B (1991). Pharyngeal flap surgery in adults. Cleft Palate-Craniofacial Journal 28(2): 179–183.

Hardin MA, Van Demark DR, Morris HL and Payne MM (1992). Correspondence between nasalance scores and listener judgements of hypernasality and hyponasality. Cleft Palate-Craniofacial Journal 29(4): 346–351.

Harrison RJ (1969). A demonstrated project of speech training for the pre-school cleft palate child: Final report. Project No. 6-1167. US Office of Education, Bureau of the Handicapped, HEW 1969.

Jarvis BL and Trier WC (1988). The effect of intravelar veloplasty on velopharyngeal competence following pharyngeal flap surgery. Cleft Palate Journal 25(4): 389 - 394.

Jenson BL, Kreiborg S, Dahl E and Fogh-Andersen P (1988). Cleft lip and palate in Denmark, 1976–1981: Epidemiology, variability and early somatic development. Cleft Palate Journal 25: 258.

Kawano M, Isshiki N, Harita Y and Tanokuchi F (1985). Laryngeal fricative in cleft palate speech. Acta Otolaryngolica 419: 180–188.

Kummer AW, Curtis C, Wiggs M, Lee L and Strife JL (1992). Comparison of velopharyngeal gap size in patients with hypernasality, hypernasality and nasal emission, or nasal turbulence (rustle) as the primary speech characteristic. Cleft Palate-Craniofacial Journal 29(2): 152–155.

Laine T, Warren DW, Dalston RM, Hairfield WM and Morr KE (1988). Intraoral pressure, nasal pressure and airflow rate in cleft palate speech. Journal of Speech and Hearing Research 31(3): 432–437.

Lynch JI, Fox DR and Brookshire BL (1988). Discontinuity in mother-child conversations: Cleft palate child compared to normal sibling. Folio Phoniatrica 40: 209–217.

McWilliams BJ (1981). Communication problems associated with cleft palate. In: Van Hattum RJ (Ed) Communication Disorders:An Introduction, 379. New York: MacMillan.

McWilliams BJ and Matthews HP (1979). A comparison of intelligence and social maturity in children with unilateral complete clefts and those with isolated cleft palates. Cleft Palate Journal 16: 363.

McWilliams BJ, Morris HL and Shelton RL (1990). Cleft Palate Speech. Philadelphia, PA: Decker.

McWilliams BJ, Glaser ER, Philips BJ and Lawrence C (1981). In: Lavorato AS, Eery BC, Skolmick ML (Eds) A Comparative Study of Four Methods Evaluating Velopharyngeal Adequacy. Plastic Reconstructive Surgery 68: 1–9.

Michi K, Suzuki N, Yamashita Y and Imai S (1986). Visual training and correction of articulation disorders by use of dynamic palatography: Serial observation in a case of cleft palate. Journal of Speech and Hearing Disorders 51: 226–238.

Morley ME (1970). Cleft Palate and Speech, (7th Edition). Baltimore MD: Williams and Wilkins.

Moss ALH, Pigott RW and Jones KJ (1988). Submucous cleft palate. British Medical Journal 297: 85–86.

Musgrave RH, McWilliams BJ and Matthews HP (1975). A review of the results of two different surgical procedures for the repair of clefts of the soft palate only. Cleft Palate Journal 12: 281–285.

Nellis JL, Neiman GS and Lehman JA (1992). Comparison of nasometer and listener judgements of nasality in the assessment of velopharyngeal function after pharyngeal flap surgery. Cleft Palate-Craniofacial Journal 29(2): 157–163.

O'Gara M and Logemann J. (1985) Acoustic assessment of the prelinguistic and linguistic vocalisations of cleft palate infants. Paper presented at the 5th International Congress on Cleft Palate and Related Craniofacial Abnormalities, Monte Carlo.

Ovesen T and Blegvad-Andersen O (1992). Alterations in tympanic membrane appearance and middle ear function in eleven-year-old children with complete unilateral cleft lip and palate compared with healthy age-matched subjects. Clinical Otolaryngology 17(3): 203–207.

Philips BJ (1979). Stimulating syntactic and phonological development in infants with cleft palate. In: Bzoch KR (Ed) Communication Disorders Related to Cleft Lip and Palate, (2nd Edition), 304. Boston, MA: Little, Brown.

Powers GR, Dunn C and Erickson CB (1990). Speech analyses of four children with repaired cleft palates. Journal of Speech and Hearing Disorders 55(3): 542–549.

Prins D and Bloomer HH (1965). The word intelligibility approach to the study of speech change in oral cleft patients. Cleft Palate Journal 2: 357.

Robinson PJ, Lodge S, Jones B, Walker C and Grant H (1992). The effect of palate repair on otitis media with effusion. Journal of Plastic and Reconstructive Surgery 89: 640–645.

Ross RB (1987). Treatment variables affecting facial growth in complete unilateral cleft lip and palate. Cleft Palate Journal 24: 5.

Schendel LL and Bzoch KR (1970). Advantages of intensive summer training programmes. In: Bzoch KR (Ed) Communicative Disorders Related to Cleft Lip and Palate. Boston, MA: Little, Brown.

Sell S (1994). Personal Communication.

Shelton RL and Ruscello DM (1979). Palatal and articulation training in patients with velopharyngeal closure problems. Annual Meeting of the American Cleft Palate Association, San Diego, CA.

Skolnick ML and McCall GN (1973). The sphincteric mechanism of velopharyngeal closure. ASHA May.

Smith JK (1969). Contra-indications for speech therapy for cleft palate speakers. Cleft Palate Journal 6: 202.

Spauwen PHM, Goorhuis-Brouwer SM and Schutte HK (1992). Cleft palate repair: Furlow versus von Langenbeck. Journal of Cranio-Maxill-Facial Surgery 20(1): 18–20.

Spriestersbach DC, Dickson DR, Fraser FC, Horowitz SL, McWilliams BJ, Paradise JL and Randall P (1973). Clinical research in cleft lip and cleft palate: the state of the art. Cleft Palate Journal 10: 113–165.

Starr CD, Moller KT, Dawson W, Graham J and Skaar S (1984). Speech ratings by speech clinicians, parents and children. Cleft Palate Journal 21(4): 286–292.

Strauss RP, Broder H and Helms RW (1988). Perceptions of appearance and speech by adolescent patients with cleft lip and palate and by their parents. Cleft Palate Journal 25(4): 335–342.

Van Demark DR (1974). Some results of speech therapy for children with cleft palate. Cleft Palate Journal 11: 41–49.

Van Demark DR and Hardin MA (1986). Effectiveness of intensive articulation therapy for children with cleft palate. Cleft Palate Journal 23: 215.

Van Demark DR, Gnoinski W, Hotz M, Perko M and Nussbaumer H (1989). Speech results of the Zurich approach in the treatment of unilateral cleft lip and palate. Plastic and Reconstructive Surgery 83(4): 605–613.

Velasco MG, Ysunza A, Hernandez X and Marquez C (1988). Diagnosis and treatment of submucous cleft palate: A review of 108 cases. Cleft Palate Journal 25(2): 171–173.

Warren DW, Dalston RM and Dalston ET (1990). Maintaining speech pressures in the presence of velopharyngeal impairment. Cleft Palate Journal 27(1): 53–58.

Wasserman GA, Allen R, and Linares LO (1988). Maternal interaction and language development in children with and without speech-related anomalies. Journal of Communication Disorders 21: 319–331.

Weatherley White RC, Sakura CY, Brenner ID, Stewart JM and Ott JE (1972). Submucous cleft palate: incidence natural history and implications for treatment. Plastic Reconstructive Surgery 49: 279.

Wells CG (1971). Cleft Palate and Its Associated Speech Disorders. New York: McGraw-Hill.

Witzell MA (1990). Craniofacial anomalies. Seminars in Speech and Language 11(3): 145–156.

Wu J, Chen YR and Noordhoff MS (1988). Articulation proficiency and error pattern of cleft palate children with delayed hard palate closure. The Annals of Academy of Medicine, Singapore 17(3): 384–387.

Young EH (1928). Overcoming Cleft Palate Speech. Minneapolis: The Hill Young School.

Zajac DJ and Linville RN (1989). Voice perturbations of children with perceived nasality and hoarseness. Cleft Palate Journal 26(3): 226–231.

Chapter 5
Dysarthria

Introduction

The term dysarthria has traditionally been defined as a disorder of speech resulting from lesions within the nervous system (Arnold, 1965). Over the years the concept of dysarthria has become more comprehensive and refined encompassing disorders beyond that just of articulation. For example, Darley, Aronson and Brown (1975) state that 'Dysarthria comprises a group of speech disorders resulting from disturbances in muscular control due to impairment of any of the basic motor processes involved in the execution of speech'. The term is now generally restricted to neurogenic speech dysfunctions resulting from impairment of the central or peripheral nervous system, including disruptions to speech related to neuromotor respiratory disorders. Frequently the term 'motor speech disorder' is used synonymously with dysarthria, however the definition of dysarthria usually excludes speech disorders of an organic/structural or of psychological origin.

Dysarthria can range in severity from a disorder so mild that it is just noticeable during rapid speech, to a disorder so severe that no functional speech is present. Frequently the latter is termed 'anarthria'.

Prevalence

Dysarthria is present in approximately 33% of all patients with traumatic brain injuries (Sarno *et al.*, 1986); 8% of individuals with cerebral palsy (Hopkins *et al.*, 1954); and varies from 19% to 100% in individuals with degenerative neurological diseases such as multiple sclerosis, Parkinson's disease and motor-neurone disease (Darley, 1978; Darley *et al.*, 1972; Logemann and Fisher, 1981).

Speech and Language Therapy for Dysarthria

Dysarthria often results in an abnormal quality of speech and reduced intelligibility. These can lead to difficulties with social interaction and limit educational and employment opportunities. Yorkston, Beukelman and Traynor (1984) note that improving speech intelligibility is the primary clinical goal with severe dysarthric speakers. This may lead the therapist to integrate augmentative communication systems into the therapy programme. For milder dysarthric speakers, the goal may shift to improving the speech quality and naturalness whilst maintaining intelligibility (Yorkston *et al.*, 1988; Yorkston *et al.*, 1990).

Despite being the most common of the acquired speech and language disorders it has attracted relatively little attention in the literature regarding its physiological and acoustic basis (Kent *et al.*, 1992), and method of assessment and treatment, or the evaluation of these. This is probably related to the fact that acquired dysarthria is frequently associated with either severe brain damage or with progressive neurological disease and there has, in the past, been a negative attitude to the role of therapy in these areas. There is some evidence that attitudes are changing and that doctors and therapists are more aware of the broad nature of rehabilitation with these disorders.

Methods of treatment for dysarthria can be crudely divided into four types (Fukusako *et al.*, 1989; Netsell, 1991).

1. A physiological approach to the impaired speech mechanism (proprioceptive neuromuscular facilitation, sensory training, muscle strengthening, etc).
2. Speech therapy for basic motor speech processes (articulation-resonance, prosody, phonation, etc).
3. Applications of instrumentation, including intraoral appliances, amplification, and bio-feedback.
4. Use of augmentative communication systems to support verbal communication or be a substitute for it, e.g. amplifiers, signing systems, hi-tech communication aids.

Efficacy of Therapy for Dysarthria Associated with Parkinson's Disease

The group of dysarthric patients which has attracted most attention regarding studies into the effectiveness of speech and language therapy are those with Parkinson's disease. The dysarthria associated with this disorder is frequently termed hypokinetic dysarthria, and is characterized by reduced articulatory range, reduced variability in pitch, stress and rhythm, reduced phonation and an increase in speaking rate. The phrasing of speech may also be disrupted.

There was a negative attitude regarding the efficacy of speech and language therapy for Parkinson's disease in the 1960s and 1970s, but more recently, a more positive attitude is reflected in the literature. Early attempts to improve the communication of these patients showed disappointing results as the improvement in treatment sessions did not seem to generalize. A rather simplistic view of dysarthria, its treatment and the measures for demonstrating its efficacy were reflected in the studies at that time. For example, a study by Sarno (1968) reviewing 300 Parkinson's patients reported that speech only improved during the treatment session and Allan (1970) reported rapid deterioration in speech following the cessation of formal speech therapy.

Contemporary speech therapy approaches utilized with Parkinsonian patients include many different approaches: delayed auditory feedback (Downie *et al.*, 1981; Low and Lindsay, 1979; Rosenbek *et al.*, 1976), the Helm Pacing Board (Helm, 1979), proprioceptive neuromuscular facilitation (Scott and Caird 1981), prosodic therapy (Scott and Caird, 1983), and intensive residential therapy (Robertson and Thomson, 1984).

Therapy involvement with this client group has radically altered since the 1980s with a much broader involvement by the therapist attempting to overcome the problems with generalizing the skills learned in therapy. More intensive treatment programmes, the involvement of relatives and follow-up support groups have attempted to improve the outcomes. However, objective evaluation of the effects of speech therapy in Parkinson's disease can still be difficult. In a paper reviewing the effectiveness of speech and language therapy, Weiner and Singer (1989) report that efficacy may not be possible to establish because 'of the fluctuating pharmacologic effect but also because improvement thought to be secondary to speech therapy may, in fact, be due to psychological factors'. This is a strange statement, as speech and language therapy from the early 1980s and in some instances prior to this has emphasized the importance of attending to psychological aspects of the disease to assist enhanced general communication.

Robertson and Thomson (1984) in a study of 22 patients, reported that intensive speech therapy programmes (group sessions plus individual sessions lasting 3.5 to 4.0 h per day for 2 weeks) had a positive affect on speech in Parkinson's disease and that some of these effects lasted for up to 3 months. The therapy aimed to improve control of respiration, coordination and control of voice production with emphasis on pitch variation and loudness, improvement of articulatory movement, control of rate of speech and intelligibility of communication. Of the 22 patients who entered the study, 12 patients were randomly allocated to a treatment group and 10 were allocated to a control group and received no therapy. Six of the control group and all 12 of the treatment group were available for follow-up assessments. The follow-up assessments showed significant improvement in the treated group with no change in the control group on all the motor speech tasks. The authors suggest that the improved insight of the patients and relatives into the disorders helped them not only to maintain a level of control, but to demonstrate further improvement after a period of 3 months without therapeutic intervention.

Scott and Caird (1981, 1983) demonstrated similar favourable benefits after a speech and language therapy treatment programme consisting of one daily session in the patient's home for 2–3 weeks. Along with the motor speech tasks, efforts were made to support and encourage patients. The positive effects were said to regress after treatment but some benefit was still detectable 3 months later. Interestingly, family members supported the conclusion that social benefits were achieved in this programme. These same authors followed this work with a further study looking at the responses of the apparent receptive speech disorder of Parkinson's Disease to speech therapy (Scott and Caird, 1984).

In an unpublished study (Johnson, 1987), and in a later study (Johnson and Pring, 1990), of a therapy approach more commonly available to patients, i.e. attending a hospital clinic once a week, two groups of patients with Parkinson's Disease were matched for age and sex; one group received a course of speech therapy whereas the other acted as controls. The assessments carried out pre and post-treatment were chosen to reflect the degree of the dysarthria, as well as the specific quantitative aspects of vocal pitch and vocal loudness. Results showed a significant improvement in overall dysarthria for the treated group. The most marked benefits were seen in the area of vocal loudness. Unfortunately this study did not have a follow-up period.

A detailed single subject multiple-baseline technique was used to investigate a programme of therapy for a 74-year-old woman presenting with Parkinson's disease. This French lady had had Parkinson's disease for about 12 years and her speech was very severely affected. The therapists reporting the case (Dorze et al., 1992) used bio-feedback (Speech Viewer System) to increase the range of fundamental frequency, to adjust the fundamental frequency to be more appropriate for her age and sex, and to modify the speaking rate. The results showed a significant change in intelligibility and in all the acoustic measures targeted: 'The patient's improvement appeared to be directly related to the treatment, i.e. the improvement occurred when attention was given to a particular speech characteristic.' The patient required 25 therapy sessions to reach the goal set and the benefits were sustained after a 10 week period of no treatment.

In describing the role of the sub-cortical structures and the thalamus in the speech mechanism, Barbeau (1969) and Botez and Barbeau (1971) concluded that speech initiation, maintenance of speech fluency and volume, control of the articulation process, and the motor pattern of the word; involved:

the periaquaductal grey matter, VL nucleus, cortical area 24, supplementary motor area, the striatum, and possibly the hypothalamus. Many investigators have deduced that a change in symptomology may be obtained by neuro-pharmacologic intervention designed to affect the neuro-chemical substrates underlying these pathways but the effect of Levodopa on dysarthria in Parkinson's disease has been inconsistent.

Nakano, Zubick and Tyler (1973) reported a significant increase in speech intelligibility after Levodopa therapy, however, other investigators found no beneficial effect (Perry and Dast, 1980; Rigordsky and Morrison, 1971).

Amantadine and anticholinergic drugs have not been found to produce a noticeable improvement in speech (Critchley 1981; Millac et al., 1970), but other drugs, such as Clonazepam, are suggested to be effective in the management of Parkinsonian dysarthria. However, Biary, Pimental and Langenberg (1988), say that the drug dosage is extremely sensitive and in a study of 12 Parkinsonian patients in a double blind trial they found that of the 11 patients who completed the study 10 showed improvement. The effective dosage of Clonazepam was found to be 0.25 to 0.5mg/d with the higher dosage than that being less effective and causing more difficulties.

Dysarthria therapy for Parkinson's disease has evolved over the past three decades. Articulation exercises, syllabic speech, chewing therapy and metronome therapy, were all used in isolation, as well as together initially, to see whether they could have an impact upon intelligibility. More recently, a more holistic approach to therapy has evolved with therapists not only concentrating on varying the acoustic aspects of the speech and vocal paucity but also endeavouring to influence posture, respiration, vocal control, pacing, phrasing and intelligibility enhancement. Different information regarding the disorder can be gained from instrumental and acoustic studies (Chenery et al., 1988; Chenery et al., 1990; Lethlean et al., 1990). Evaluative studies rarely report on both. Furthermore, therapists are more aware of the psychological impact and the importance of engaging the patient's insight so that they can assist with controlling their own symptoms (Morley, 1990). Associated impairments affecting communication are only recently becoming understood, e.g. receptive disorders and negative affect (Scott and Caird, 1984).

Given that the dysarthria associated with Parkinson's disease is common, there is a need for more basic research into different therapeutic programmes and into investigating the efficacy of the combinations of the different packages.

A detailed and considered review of the literature relating to speech therapy and Parkinson's Disease, by Johnson and Pring (1990), concludes that the immediate gains from therapy measured within the clinical setting are readily detected and that these benefits persist for some period after treatment.

Speech and Language Therapy for Severe Dysarthria

There have been a series of single case reports explaining the role and the outcomes for speech therapy with severely dysarthric patients. These are difficult to amalgamate as the aetiologies are different, but they have some common features which lead them to be grouped together for the purpose of this review.

A detailed case study (Simpson *et al.*., 1988) describing the long-term treatment and changing symptoms in a single subject with dysarthria secondary to basilar artery thrombosis, details the course of this subject from totally anarthric and 'locked-in' to the position 3 years later where he was having a degree of functional oral communication. The gains were slow over the 3 year period. The speech therapy was not intensive but was described as being 'essential in leading the programme of care by targeting efforts in a structured way'. The foci of therapy were directed towards modifying speech respiration, velopharyngeal function, articulatory precision, speech intensity and speech intelligibility. A variety of treatment measurement techniques were illustrated using bio-feedback and other devices. Although gains on each of the parameters were small, these gains when combined, were reported as resulting 'in improved communication and quality of life'. The therapy was multi-faceted. The therapists involved monitored and developed an augmenta-tive communication system appropriate to the circumstances throughout the course of the 3 years. They developed an 'abdominal' binder to support respiration and used visual feedback to encourage improvement in vital capacity and vocal control. Intraoral appliances were used to improve the closure of the velopharynx and an amplifier was introduced to reduce effort. The range of skills required in treat-ment and the benefits that these had for this client are well demon-strated in this paper.

This modular approach is also emphasized in a case study used to illustrate speech rehabilitation of a 20-year-old unintelligible man who had severe flaccid dysarthria following head injury (Netsell and Daniel, 1979). These authors similarly emphasized the selection and sequencing of treatment procedures for severely dysarthric patients, arguing that these are 'conditioned by the inherent physical inter-dependencies of component parts'. In this case, respiratory therapy, along with improve-ments of the velopharynx were concentrated on for the first 3 weeks. These included manometry and intraoral appliances. From the third to the fifth week, concentration was on the laryngeal area with bio-feed-back to improve vocal control. The oral facial aspect was not attended to until the last 2 weeks of the 6 week period of treatment. This patient had previously received speech therapy of a more general nature and the authors suggest that his improvement, which is plotted in the paper, was related to the structured approach to therapy. On discharge, this client's speech was rated as 95% intelligible and although his voice was somewhat breathy and nasal, the loudness was only slightly reduced. Results, 3 years after discharge from treatment, reveal that he had maintained the intelligibility and his speech and voice had further improved. By that time, this man had returned to employment.

Some 25 years after a head injury, a 30 year old subject was treated for his severe dysarthria (Hartman *et al.*, 1979). This patient had a long-standing severe dysarthria and had not received previous therapy. The treatment programme detailed in the paper follows the Darley approach (Darley, 1978). Work on improving his articulation and to maximize the remaining potential, along with teaching a sign system to accompany speech and emphasis on developing his own personal auditory monitoring, apparently resulted in feedback which generalized to non-trained aspects of communication. Unfortunately this paper, along with many others, is descriptive and does not give sufficient detail to analyse specific results.

A similar report, reviewing the progress of four ataxic dysarthric speakers, demonstrates again the general consensus that speech and language therapy, for this group of patients, is multi-faceted and sequential (Yorkston and Beukelman, 1981). The four subjects exhibited sudden onset of ataxic dysarthria. Two cases were related to encephalopathy and two cases to head injury. A hierarchy of rate control strategies, ranging from rigid imposition of rate through rhythmic cuing, to self-monitored rate control, is discussed. As speakers improved their monitoring skills, a compromise was made between intelligibility and rate. Normal prosodic patterns were not achieved by the ataxic speakers due to difficulty in precisely coordinating the subtle fundamental frequency, loudness and timing adjustments needed to signal prosodic stress. Three of the four subjects were taught to use only durational adjustments to signal stress. The authors conclude, that, while many principles have been drawn from clinical practice, they feel that research is necessary to verify and refine these approaches. They give the example of rate control strategies which have received little attention. Clinical judgements preferring one rate control strategy over another are made without a clear understanding of the consequences of these strategies on other aspects of speech.

The timing of intervention with severely head-injured patients also needs to be reviewed. Four subjects with severe dysarthria and profound physical disability following head injury were monitored for 7 years by Enderby and Crow (1990); all were assessed using the same assessment at regular intervals. Despite the fact that the subjects remained severely dysarthric and used communication aids, oral motor improvements have been detected and are argued to have functional relevance. A few gains were noted in the first 18 months, but one subject only showed improvement after 24 months post incident, another subject after 30 months, with the most substantial changes for all subjects being seen by 48 months post injury. Further small improvements continued to be recorded up until the end of the study.

A case study, which is stated by the authors not to be 'research' but 'the report of a clinical service', details the 10 year speech therapy programme for a young man with severe dysarthria associated with Wilson's disease. Initially, he was classified as being '100% disabled', but eventually he was able to secure full-time employment, which required some degree of verbal communication. The authors argue that this case does suggest that long-term therapy might be worthy of consideration and cost effective as an option for some carefully selected dysarthric clients. They feel it is essential that the client is actively involved in the evaluation of his own speech; attention to general guidelines is more effective than work on specific phonemic aspects of speech production to assist generalization; the use of systematic probes to assess intelligibility in situations external to the clinical setting; and the incorporation of feedback from conversational partners (Day and Parnell, 1987).

The only large group study published recently, which evaluated the efficacy of speech and language therapy for dysarthria associated with stroke, was reported by Fukusako *et al*. (1989). This follows the course of 24 dysarthric patients and combines single case studies and group results. The ages, severity of speech disorder and associated difficulties, are various. This, along with the very diverse therapy, makes it difficult to interpret the results. However, the authors report an improvement in severity (the sum of the scale values of bizarreness and intelligibility) for 16 of the 24 patients and a prominent improvement was noted for seven patients. They concluded that the more profoundly that speech performance was impaired before treatment, the more improvement was obtained. Not surprisingly there was a considerable variability in the degree and type of improvement.

Speech and Language Therapy for Mild Dysarthria

Phrasing

Mildly dysarthric speakers frequently form a challenge to speech and language therapists as their speech can be intelligible but bizarre or monotonous. Bellaire, Yorkston and Beukelman (1986) investigated the case of a 20-year-old closed-head injured man, with mild dysarthria, and examined different ways of increasing the naturalness of speech with respiratory control. They judged that the difficulties resulted from short uniform breath groups and inhalation during every pause, along with restricted fundamental frequency range. They sought to train the patient to improve in the first two of these factors. The patient was able to learn to vary the length of the breath group and to use pausing as a strategy to chunk speech.

This study, along with others, causes some difficulty when one is considering true outcome measures of dysarthria therapy. If the outcome is for the patient to achieve speech similar to normal, then it is likely that the results of efficacy studies would be different from if one chose the outcome to be speech which is more intelligible or less bizarre. Frequently a patient is taught to speak in a more abnormal way so that his or her speech is more intelligible, e.g slowing down speaking rate to that well below normal. In addition it is possible to learn ways of using stress and breathing to give the appearance of greater fluency. These almost trick the listener into the feeling that speech is more normal.

Intelligibility enhancement

The methodological difficulties of selecting appropriate outcome measures is further complicated by considering the aspects which affect intelligibility. Some studies do not explain how intelligibility ratings are achieved and there is evidence that intelligibility can be affected by many different conditions. An example of this is found in a study designed to determine whether the use of the aided speech technique (the patient points to the first letter of each word on the alphabet chart as he speaks the word), described by Beukelman and Yorkston (1977), changes the auditory characteristics of speech, thereby improving the speech intelligibility of dysarthric speakers, or whether it is the visual clue that assists the listener to interpret. In this study, six speakers with dysarthria were examined under two conditions (Enderby and Crow, 1989). In the first they spoke habitually and in the second condition they pointed to the first letter of each word on an alphabet chart before saying the word. Audio recordings of the speech samples were then played to a group of listeners. Measures of intelligibility and speaking rate were made along with phonetic transcription. When speakers used the alphabet chart to aid their speech, it was found that intelligibility increased, speaking rate decreased and articulatory accuracy improved as compared with habitual speech.

Hunter, Pring and Martin (1991) investigated the effects of strategies on the intelligibility of cerebral palsied speech. Listeners were asked to interpret words spoken by moderate or severely dysarthric persons. The speech samples were presented under four conditions: auditory only, auditory plus visual, auditory plus visual with repetition, and auditory plus initial letter cuing. An experimental design was used and demonstrated that different strategies increased intelligibility and that different strategies had different effects for different levels of severity of dysarthria. The use of initial letter cuing achieved the greatest gains for the more severely impaired speakers; but for the less severely impaired, gains achieved by providing visual cues were the same as those achieved by letter cuing and could not be improved upon by repetition.

Listeners experience of dysarthric speech and the redundancy of the test sentence were also manipulated. Although previous experience did not influence the recognition, redundancy appeared to have an influence at higher levels of intelligibility only. Thus, different strategies are appropriate for different severities of dysarthria in assisting the listener to pick up on what is being said. These strategies are frequently used in order to support assist or prompt the listener, rather than to modify the spoken output of a patient. At present the limited research in this field has not taken account of some of these complicated outcome parameters (Ansel and Kent, 1992).

Feedback

There is evidence that a speaker, realising the listener is not able to understand, will adjust speech accordingly. Such adjustments may be by raising the volume, slowing the speaking rate and re-phrasing utterances.

Most of the studies have reported modifications in language output made by children when they realise they are failing to communicate. Till and Toye (1988) studied the effects of two different forms of verbal feedback on changes in the speech production of seven dysarthric speakers. Both forms of feedback indicated to the speaker that the listener had failed to understand the message. One form was of a general nature and gave no specific clues regarding the reason why the listener had failed to understand. The other gave more specific information.

The subject's response showed a significant change in the specific area of failure, i.e. voice onset time (VOT), after the specific feedback and no significant change in VOT after the more general feedback.

It appears from this that the use of specific feedback to induce articulatory change which results in improved intelligibility is warranted. As with many of the studies on dysarthria, the reader lacks confidence as to whether the aetiology of the dysarthria is correctly identified.

Instrumental forms of feedback have been used in a number of studies. A report using delayed auditory feedback to assist in the treatment of a 59-year-old male, with progressive supra-nuclear palsy, is a good example (Hanson and Metter, 1980). This subject had a hypokinetic dysarthria which had not responded to therapy prior to being introduced to a small, delayed auditory feedback device which was used to reduce speaking rate and aid speech intelligibility. The patient wore the device, on a daily basis, for 3 months. Measure of speech rate, intensity and overall intelligibility indicated that when the instrument was worn, the subjects speech was slowed, intensity increased and intelligibility markedly improved. The subject and his family reported satisfaction with the instrument. This paper was presented in 1980. Despite this, the use of delayed auditory feedback as a continual aid to intelligibility is very rarely tried in clinical practice.

The same authors report the beneficial effects of the same device with two patients with Parkinson's disease, one making much greater gains than the other (Hanson and Metter, 1983). Delayed auditory feedback does require some degree of tolerance and cooperation on the part of the patient and therefore it is possible that, despite the positive effects upon control in volume and fluency, there may be some user resistance.

In order to assess the effectiveness of a computer-based speech training system (CBST), Thomas-Stonell, McClean and Hunt (1991) evaluated the effectiveness of the IBM Speech Viewer CBST combined with a newly developed rate control programme for improving speech production in individuals with dysarthria. Three subjects were studied using a single subject multiple baseline design. Voice timing, speaking rate, and vowel accuracy were trained sequentially. Dependent measures included: speech intelligibility, speaking rate and acoustic measures obtained on selected speech parameters. Four of the six multiple baseline treatment phases revealed significant training effects. The other two phases revealed trends towards normal values. There was a total of eight multiple baseline treatment phases across the three subjects, but six of these were analysed statistically. The three subjects were of different ages, 18 years, 17 years and 5 years old, with different aetiologies, head injury and myotonic dystrophy. Different information is reported for the different patients and it is difficult to know whether only the positive gains are reported in this paper. For example, it is reported that subject number one continued some carry-over 6 months after the completion of the study, but the carry-over results of the other two are not referred to.

Achieving generalizability of speech gains outside the clinic motivated Rubow and Swift (1985) to develop a microcomputer-based wearable biofeedback device. This monitored and fed-back information on vocal intensity and in the reported case study was successful in maintaining speech performance of one Parkinsonian subject at 10 and 20 weeks post-treatment follow-up.

It has been noted that immediate and accurate visual feedback can assist in training motor tasks. This is very likely to be the case in speech disorders. The feedback from therapists may be neither timely nor accurate and is, of course, absent when a therapist is not with the patient. By providing accurate visual feedback, patients can improve their own ability to monitor their speaking behaviour. The hypotheses as to whether this assists the patient to speak more accurately, and that this generalizes to speech tasks not being monitored, have been tested by a few authors (Berry and Goshorn, 1983). Although the number of studies reported are small and most describe one or two subjects, the results all seem to indicate that this form of approach, in therapy, is efficacious.

Prosthetic intervention

Hypernasality caused by palatal insufficiency is a common feature with many dysarthric patients. The management of hypernasality either by using bio-feedback or prosthesis has attracted some attention within the literature. It is now generally considered that prosthetic intervention is effective with a select group of dysarthrics. The appliances consist of a plate that covers the hard palate and is attached to the teeth. If the patient wears a denture then the appliance can be attached to that. Attached to the rear of the plate is an extension of acrylic shaped to fit the patient's oropharynx. This pushes the palate up and back providing improved closure of the nasopharyngeal opening. There is consensus that patients with the following characteristics are the best candidates for palatal lift prosthesis: those who are extremely hypernasal and whose soft palates and pharyngeal muscles are not spastic, and patients who have teeth, or a very good fitting denture, to which the prosthesis can be anchored (Netsell and Rosenbek, 1985; Rosenbek and La Pointe, 1985; Yorkston *et al.*, 1988). Patients who have reasonably good articulation and phonation and where hypernasality is one of the main characteristics, appear to do particularly well. Obviously patients have to be cooperative but it has been suggested, by these authors, that those who have swallowing difficulties may not do so well as those without such problems.

A case report by Brand, Matsko and Avart (1988) described the treatment using a speech prosthesis, of a 20-year-old woman who had difficulty in retaining the appliance. The therapists in this case persisted because speech intelligibility was maximized via the fitting of the intraoral appliance. The case reports overcoming the retention problems by using a topical anaesthetic as the traditional desensitization techniques were unsuccessful.

A report of 37 dysarthric patients with velopharyngeal insufficiency, who were treated with a palatal lift prosthesis (Michi *et al.*, 1988), indicated that speech intelligibility improved significantly (i.e. by more than 10%) in 15 patients, slightly in three patients, remained unchanged in 13 and deteriorated in two. Suggestions regarding the selection of patients support the indications mentioned previously.

Conclusion

Dysarthria is the most commonly acquired speech and language disorder. Additionally, it is not an uncommon developmental disorder. There has been considerable effort in describing the neurological basis and the acoustic effects of this disorder, and there appears to be general consensus regarding the hypotheses suggested in these areas (Kent *et al.*, 1992; Solomon and Hixon, 1993; Ziegler *et al.*, 1993). However, there are relatively few texts detailing the therapeutic approaches suitable for the different speech impairments but those that have been recently published make up in quality for what is lacked in quantity. The serious omissions in the area regarding dysarthria efficacy relate to the inadequate development of outcome measures for the disorder, for example, many studies use specific speech analysis techniques such as spectroanalysis etc, whereas, other features of the speech may not be reported upon.

Research into the efficacy of speech and language therapy for dysarthria is greatly hampered by the lack of standardized methods of assessing the overall effects of the disorder. Furthermore, the majority of the few efficacy studies lack sufficient detail regarding the aetiology of the dysarthria to make them useful. There have been no studies that we have come across that have looked at the effects of dysarthria in a more general way, for example, the psychosocial effects of the impairment. Seeing that a considerable amount of speech and language therapy appears to be targeted on the psychosocial aspects, it is surprising that so little emphasis on this is made in the efficacy literature.

References

Allan CM (1970). Treatment of non-fluent speech resulting from neurological disease: Treatment of dysarthria. British Journal of Disorders of Communication 5: 3–5.

Ansel BM and Kent RD (1992). Acoustic-phonetic contrasts and intelligibility in the dysarthria associated with mixed cerebral palsy. Journal of Speech and Hearing Research 35: 296–308.

Arnold GE (1965). Central nervous disorders of speaking: Dysarthria. In: Luchsinger R and Arnold GE (Eds) Voice, Speech, Language. Belmont: Wadsworth.

Barbeau A (1969). L-Dopa therapy in Parkinson's disease: A critical review of nine years' experience. Canadian Medical Association Journal 101: 59–68.

Bellaire K, Yorkston KM and Beukelman D (1986). Modification of breath patterning to increase naturalness of a mildly dysarthric speaker. Journal of Communication Disorders 19: 271 -280.

Berry WR and Goshorn EL (1983). Immediate visual feedback in the treatment of ataxic dysarthria: A case study. In: Berry WR (Ed) Clinical Dysarthria. San Diego, CA: College Hill Press.

Beukelman D and Yorkston K (1977). A communication system for severely dysarthric speakers with an intact language system. Journal of Speech and Hearing Disorders 42: 265–266.

Biary N, Pimental P and Langenberg P (1988). A double blind trial of clonazepam in the treatment of Parkinsonian dysarthria. Neurology 38: 255–258.

Botez MI and Barbeau A (1971). Role of sub-cortical structures and particularly of the thalamus, in the mechanisms of speech and language. International Journal of Neurology 8: 300–320.

Brand H, Matsko TA and Avart HN (1988). Speech prosthesis retention problems in dysarthria: Case report: Archives of Physical Medicine and Rehabilitation 69: 213–214.

Chenery HJ, Murdoch BE and Ingram JC (1988). Studies in Parkinson's disease: Perceptual speech analysis. Australian Journal of Human Communication Disorders 16(2): 17–29.

Chenery HJ, Ingram JC and Murdoch BE (1990). Perceptual analysis of the speech in ataxic dysathria. Australian Journal of Human Communication Disorders 18: 19–27.

Critchley EM (1981). Speech disorders of Parkinsonism: A review. Journal of Neurology, Neurosurgery and Psychiatry 44: 751–758.

Darley FL (1978). Differential diagnosis of acquired motor speech disorders. In: Darley FL and Spriestersbach DC (Eds) Diagnostic Methods in Speech Pathology (2nd Edition) New York: Harper and Row.

Darley FL, Brown JR and Goldstein NP (1972). Dysarthria in multiple sclerosis. Journal of Speech and Hearing Research 15: 229–245.

Darley FL, Aronson AE and Brown JR (1975). Motor Speech Disorders. Philadelphia, PA: WB Saunders.

Day LS and Parnell MM (1987). Ten year study of a Wilson's disease dysarthric. Journal of Communication Disorders 20: 207–218.

Dorze G, Dionne L, Ryalls J, Julien M and Ouellet L (1992). The effects of speech and language therapy for a case of dysarthria associated with Parkinson's disease. The European Journal of Disorders of Communication 27: 313–324.

Downie A, Low JM and Lindsay O (1981). Speech disorders in Parkinsonism: Usefulness of delayed auditory feedback in selected cases. British Journal of Disorders of Communication 16: 135 -139.

Enderby P and Crow E (1989). The effects of an alphabet chart on the speaking rate and intelligibility of speakers with dysarthria. In: Yorkston K and Beukelman D (Eds) Recent Advances in Clinical Dysarthria. Boston, MA: College Hill Press.

Enderby P and Crow E (1990). Long term recovery patterns of severe dysarthria following head injury. British Journal of Disorders of Communication 25: 341–354.

Fukusako Y, Endo K, Konno K, Hasegawa K, Tatsumi I, Masaki S, Kawamura M, Shiota J and Hirose H (1989). Changes in speech of spastic dysarthric patients after treatment based on perceptual analysis. Annual Bulletin RILP 23: 119–140.

Hanson WR and Metter EJ (1980). DAF as instrumental treatment for dysarthria in progressive supra-nuclear palsy: A case report. Journal of Speech and Hearing Disorders 45: 268–276.

Hanson WR and Metter EJ (1983). DAF speech rate modification in Parkinson's disease: A report of two cases. In: Berry WR (Ed) Clinical Dysarthria. San Diego, CA: College Hill Press.

Hartman D, Day M and Pecora R (1979). Dysarthria: A single case study of head injury. Journal of Communication Disorders 12: 167–173.

Helm N (1979). Management of palilalia with a pacing board. Journal of Speech and Hearing Disorders 44: 350–353.

Hopkins T, Bice HV and Colton KC (1954). Valuation and education of the cerebral palsied child – the New Jersey study. Washington, DC: International Council for Exceptional Children.

Hunter L, Pring T and Martin S (1991). The use of strategies to increase speech intelligibility in cerebral palsy: An experimental evaluation. British Journal of Disorders of Communication 26: 163–174.

Johnson J (1987). An in-depth assessment of a short course of speech therapy in Parkinson's disease. MSc thesis, City University, London.

Johnson JH and Pring TR (1990). Speech therapy with Parkinson's disease: A review and further data. British Journal of Disorders of Communication 25: 183–194.

Kent JF, Kent RD, Rosenbek JC, Weismer G, Martin R, Sufit R and Brooks BR (1992). Quantitative description of the dysarthria in women with amyotrophic lateral sclerosis. Journal of Speech and Hearing Research 35: 723–733.

Lethlean JB, Chenery HJ and Murdoch BE (1990). Disturbed respiratory and prosodic function in Parkinson's disease: A perceptual and instrumental analysis: Australian Journal of Speech and Human Communication Disorders 18: (2) 83–97.

Logemann JA and Fisher HB (1981). Vocal tract control in Parkinson's disease: Phonetic feature analysis of mis-articulations. Journal of Speech and Hearing Disorders 46(4): 248–352.

Low J and Lindsay DD (1979). A body worn delayed auditory feedback fluency aid for stammerers. Journal of Bio-Medical Engineering 1: 235–239.

Michi K, Yamashita Y, Imai S, Arisawa Y and Suzuki N (1988). The use of palatal lift prosthesis with velopharyngeal insufficiency resulting from acquired neurological disease. Japanese Journal of Logopaedics and Phoniatrics 29: 239–255. (In Japanese)

Millac P, Hassan I, Espir M and Slyfield D (1970). Amantidine in Parkinson's disease. Lancet 1: 464.

Morley R (1990). Speech therapy and Parkinson's disease – a long term commitment. Care of the Elderly 2(2): 58–59.

Nakano KK, Zubick H and Tyler HR (1973). Speech defects of Parkinsonian patients. Neurology 23: 865–870.

Netsell R (1991). A Neurobiologic View of Speech Production and the Dysarthrias. San Diego, CA: Singular.

Netsell R and Daniel B (1979). Dysarthria in adults: Physiologic approach to rehabilitation. Archives of Physical Medicine and Rehabilitation 60: 502–508.

Netsell R and Rosenbek JC (1985). Treating the dysarthrias. In: Darby J (Ed) Speech and Language Evaluation in Neurology: Adult Disorders. New York: Grune and Stratton.

Perry AR and Dast PK (1980). Speech assessment in Parkinson's disease. In: Rose FC and Capildeo R (Eds) Research in Parkinson's Disease, 373–384. London: Pitman.

Rigordsky S and Morrison EB (1971). Speech changes in Parkinsonism during L-dopa Therapy: preliminary findings. Journal of the American Geriatric Society 18: 142–151.

Robertson SJ and Thomson F (1984). Speech therapy and Parkinson's disease: A study of the efficacy and long term affects of intensive treatment. British Journal of Disorders of Communication 19: 213–224.

Rosenbek JC and La Pointe LL (1985). The dysarthrias: Description, diagnoses, and treatment. In: Johns DF (Ed) Clinical Management of Neurogenic Communication Disorders (2nd Edition), 97–152. Boston, MA: Little, Brown.

Rosenbek JD, Wertz RT and Collins M (1976). Delayed auditory feedback in dysarthria treatment. Presentation to the American Speech and Hearing Association, Houston, TX.

Rubow R and Swift E (1985). A microcomputer-based wearable biofeedback device to improve transfer of treatment in Parkinsonian dysarthria. Journal of Speech and Hearing Disorders 50: 178–185.

Sarno MT (1968). Speech impairment in Parkinson's disease. Archives of Physical Medicine and Rehabilitation 49: 269.

Sarno MT, Buonagura A and Levita E (1986). Characteristics of verbal impairment in closed head injured patients. Archives of Physical Medicine and Rehabilitation 67: 400–405.

Scott S and Caird F (1981). Speech therapy for patients with Parkinson's disease. British Medical Journal 283: 1088.

Scott S and Caird F (1983). Speech therapy for Parkinson's disease: Journal of Neurology, Neurosurgery and Psychiatry 46: 140–144.

Scott S and Caird F (1984). The response of the apparent receptive speech disorder of Parkinson's disease to speech therapy. Journal of Neurology, Neurosurgery and Psychiatry 47: 302–304.

Simpson M, Till J and Goff A (1988). Long term treatment of severe dysarthria: A case study. Journal of Speech and Hearing Disorders 53: 433–440.

Solomon NP and Hixon T (1993). Speech breathing in Parkinson's disease. Journal of Speech and Hearing Research 36: 294–693.

Thomas-Stonell N, McClean M and Hunt E (1991). Evaluation of the Speech Viewer computer-based speech training system with neurologically impaired individuals. JSLPA 15(4): 47–53.

Till JA, and Toye AR (1988). Acoustic phonetic affects of two types of verbal feedback in dysarthric subjects. Journal of Speech and Hearing Disorders 53: 449–458.

Weiner WJ, Singer C (1989). Parkinson's disease and non-pharmacologic treatment programmes. Journal of the American Geriatric Society 37(4): 359–363.

Yorkston KM and Beukelman DR (1981). Ataxic dysarthria: Treatment sequences based on intelligibility and prosodic considerations. Journal of Speech and Hearing Disorders 46: 398–404.

Yorkston K, Beukelman D and Traynor C (1984). Computerized Assessment of Intelligibility of Dysarthric Speakers. Austin, TX: Pro-Ed.

Yorkston KM, Beukelman DR and Bell KR (1988). Clinical Management of Dysarthric Speakers. San Diego, CA: College Hill Press.

Yorkston K, Hammen VL, Beukelman D and Traynor C (1990). The effect of rate control on the intelligibility and naturalness of dysarthric speech. Journal of Speech and Hearing Disorders 55(3): 550–559.

Ziegler W, Hartman E and Hoole P (1993). Syllabic timing in dysarthria. Journal of Speech and Hearing Research 36: 683–693.

Chapter 6
Laryngectomy

Introduction

Laryngectomy refers to the surgical removal of the larynx, which is primarily necessitated because of cancer within the larynx or associated areas. Occasionally laryngectomy is necessary because of trauma or other disease.

It has been estimated that there are almost 1500 people, each year, in the British Isles who suffer from cancer of the larynx. About one-third of these require total laryngectomy (Priest, 1991). The incidence and mortality rate from laryngeal cancer is reported to be rising throughout the world. There was a moderate increase in incidence reported in England and Wales throughout the 1960s. All available epidemiological evidence points to an association between tobacco use and laryngeal cancer, including a strong dose—response relationship with both the number of cigarettes smoked and the duration of the smoking habit. Alcohol has also been claimed to be a causative factor acting both alone and synergistically with cigarette smoking. It appears from this paper, that the age-standardized mortality rates for cancer in the larynx was just under 2 per 100 000 (Barclay and Rao, 1975).

The 5-year cure rate of laryngeal carcinoma with preservation of voice and glottic function is suggested by several authors to be as high as 90% as long as the lesions of the vocal cords are found at an early stage (McKenna *et al.*, 1991).

An analysis of 3445 cases of cancer of the larynx, in the United Kingdom, was made with reference to primary and secondary treatments. The findings confirmed that, while radiotherapy was inferior to laryngectomy in the cure of large glottic tumours, it was preferable in some other cases because salvage surgery was possible and successful. Salvage surgery was not shown to be successful in larger supraglottic tumours and it was recommended that these should be considered for primary surgery (Robin *et al.*, 1991).

The incidence of laryngectomy is influenced by a number of different factors, including: early detection of laryngeal tumour which relates to the astuteness of primary health care and general health education of the population; philosophies regarding radiotherapy as a primary intervention; and surgical approaches to tumour management without total laryngectomy (Boyle *et al.*, 1982).

Thus, the prevalence of laryngectomy varies, not only between countries but also, probably, within a country by geographical area. Because the number of patients undergoing laryngectomy per year is not well documented, the number of therapists required to support post-laryngectomy rehabilitation is harder to plan. It has been deduced that, within the United Kingdom, the prevalence of laryngectomy is between 0.9 and 3 per 100 000 population (Enderby and Davies, 1989).

Pathology

A total laryngectomy entails the total removal of the larynx including the hyoid bone superiorly and upper rings of the trachea inferiorly; the resulting defect in the anterior wall of the pharynx is closed by joining the edges thus creating a new food passage completely separate from the airway (Cheesman, 1983). The upper end of the trachea is brought out through the skin at the front of the neck to create a stoma. Total laryngectomy generally controls the primary tumour but, occasionally, due to involvement of the lymph nodes, a block dissection or radical neck dissection will also be required. Some patients require less extensive surgery involving partial laryngectomy, removing maybe, one part of the thyroid cartilage and vocal cord. Others will require more extensive surgery, including removal of the larynx with a part of the oesophagus and laryngo-pharynx. The possibilities and types of speech rehabilitation available to patients depends on the surgery involved. Patients requiring a transplanted part of colon or jejunum due to a pharyngolaryngooesophagectomy will need a completely different rehabilitation programme from those with partial or total laryngectomy (Ranger, 1983).

Speech and Language Therapy

Developing oesophageal communication

Oesophageal speech requires the patient to develop a method of injecting the air into the oesophagus below the pharyngo-oesophageal segment (PE segment) and being able to control this source of air to support speech. On average, the upper one-third of the oesophagus can accommodate 80 cc of air. The method of introducing air into the oesophagus was originally thought to be similar to swallowing, but this has now been disputed (Salmon, 1979).

Some patients, unable for various reasons to be able to introduce air into the oesophagus, speak on air stored in the pharynx and this speech is often termed 'buccal speech'. Patients frequently have problems in the following areas.

1. The ability to inject air.
2. The ability to control the expulsion of air.
3. Coordinating air-flow with speech.
4. Controlling the volume of oesophageal sound.
5. Controlling noise from the stoma which may mask speech clarity.
6. Ensuring that articulation maximises intelligibility.

Speech and Language therapists are frequently the professionals who assist the patient and the family to come to terms with speech impairment and its resultant disability and handicaps. Counselling is generally accepted as playing a large role in the intervention.

Whilst the psychological sequelae are recognized as frequently being devastating (Bronheim *et al.*, 1991), few studies have investigated the most efficacious ways of encouraging emotional adaptation by the patient and family. One retrospective study was able to relate enhanced psychological adaption to pre-operative teaching, post-operative rehabilitation and psychiatric intervention (Natvig, 1983a). Prospective studies assessing the effectiveness of different methods of providing support and information are lacking. Williams (1994) calls for qualitative research techniques to be used to expand our knowledge in this area.

Whilst in the United Kingdom speech rehabilitation is usually provided by speech and language therapists, this is not the case in all countries. Lehmann and Krebs (1991) conducted a patient opinion survey of 332 laryngectomees resident in Switzerland. He reports that, for the whole of Switzerland, approximately one-fifth of laryngectomees received speech training from another laryngectomee; but in the Italian-speaking part the figure was as high as 80%. The average duration of speech rehabilitation was 12 weeks; the range was from 1 week to more than 52 weeks with an average of 20 lessons. Half of the laryngectomees took 1—3 months to learn to communicate, however, 20% needed 4—6 months and 15% took even longer. Of those involved in the survey, 5% were unable to use speech as a form of communication for the interview, 65% were satisfied with their speech rehabilitation and 17% were dissatisfied.

Oesophageal speech requires control of the air reservoir by the PE segment and in more extensive surgery this is anatomically difficult. Whilst air can be injected into the transplanted colon or oesophagus constructed from skin flaps, the tone of these would be such that the resistance will be low, causing less audible and lower frequency vibration (Vize, 1976).

Artificial larynges

Laryngectomees in their immediate post-operative stage are frequently instructed to use a temporary means of communication such as writing until they can begin to learn oesophageal speech. The use of artificial larynges, neck type and intraoral have become increasingly used as an option to consider in rehabilitation. Whilst these were thought to be 'the last resort' if oesophageal speech had not been successful, the improvements in design of larynges is such, that they are now used as a primary alternative so that patients can choose different methods of communication within different environments. Most patients are now offered the option of learning to use a laryngeal artificial communication with a technological appliance in addition to the oesophageal speech.

Concern has been expressed about the acceptability of speech obtained with an artificial larynx on naive listeners. The responses of listeners to unaided alaryngeal speech and to speech using artificial larynges were studied when 30 service-station attendants were exposed to both speech patterns. The authors concluded that listener reactions should not be cited as an argument against the use of an artificial larynx as adverse reactions seemed to be minimal, were coped with easily, and did not interfere with effective communication (Hartman and Scott, 1974).

Some therapists used to have reservations about introducing appliances due to their concern that the use of an artificial larynx might impede the learning of oesophageal speech. However, Gates *et al*. (1982), after an extensive study of 53 laryngectomized patients over a 6 month period, concluded that early use of artificial larynges enhanced their patients' learning of oesophageal speech. Therapists need to be aware, not only of the technical devices available and the aspects that make one device more appropriate for one patient than another, but also the methods of maximizing the clarity and acceptability of these forms of speech. Different techniques for choosing and introducing these aids are described in the literature (Salmon, 1983), but they have not been stringently evaluated (Levy and Abramson, 1983).

Vocal prostheses

The first vocal prosthesis, which routed the air from the lungs through a tracheal segment into the nose, was described in 1873. Efforts in rehabilitation using vocal prostheses have been reported since that time; these can be subdivided on the basis of techniques employed: pharyngo-cutaneous fistula with prosthesis, internal fistula without prosthesis, electronic implants and internal fistula with prosthesis (Smith, 1982).

The objective of many of these surgical speech rehabilitation techniques is to recreate the physiological situation after the larynx has been removed so that the air expired from the lungs generates a vibration, albeit not of the vocal cords, and supports the articulation of speech sounds. By harnessing the respiratory system to voice production, one allows a more natural pacing and production of sound. The volume of air, the ease of inspiration and the more easily controllable expiration, all facilitate more natural phrasing with less effort. This has been said to offer more vocal power, fluency, flexibility and a better natural quality. The most commonly used surgical approach to speech rehabilitation presently in practice is that pioneered by Singer, Blom and Haymaker (1981). This technique creates a direct tract through the adjacent walls of trachea and oesophagus and can be used as a primary or secondary technique (Perry 1988). The pros and cons of surgical voice restoration being performed as a primary or secondary procedure are hotly debated (Radford, 1993). Small, unobtrusive, relatively inexpensive prosthetic tubes with one-way valves have been devised to prevent fluid leakage through the lumen. A survey of 100 randomly chosen otolaryngologists in the United Kingdom, resulting in a 56% response rate, recorded that the Blom-Singer valve is the most popular, being used in 35 of 44 units (79%); Provox valve 43%; and the Groningen valve was used by 5% (Parker, 1993). The therapist is not only involved in helping the person to control the phonatory air-flow through the prosthesis but also is frequently the one who teaches the patient to manage the 'puncture' and valve.

Evaluative Research

Oesophageal speech

There are a limited number of studies reviewing mortality and morbidity following laryngectomy. There are even fewer studies relating to speech outcome. Whilst there have been several retrospective studies dealing with the relationship between the extent of surgery and the ability to learn oesophageal speech, indicating that the more radical surgery leads to less good speech outcome (Richardson, 1981), there are fewer studies that look at the variables related to speech training in the development of oesophageal speech. Not surprisingly, Richardson and Bourque (1985) found that oesophageal speakers spent more time practising their speech than non oesophageal speakers. Satisfaction with speech training has been found, in some studies, to be an important predictor of oesophageal speech (Mathieson *et al.*, 1990).

Natvig (1983b), devised a scale to distinguish socially acceptable from non-acceptable oesophageal speech, and then related the resulting speech categories to time lapse from laryngectomy to the start of speech and language therapy, the number of lessons received, the satisfaction with speech lessons, and the patients first impressions of their own voice.

Only satisfaction with speech lessons was significantly related to acceptable speech in this study. Similarly, Stam, Scott and Mathieson (1990) found that satisfaction with speech training was an important predictor of the acquisition of successful oesophageal speech production.

A retrospective study of 55 laryngectomees compared the outcomes of those who received speech and language therapy as early as 2–3 weeks post-operatively with those who received therapy 1 year or more after surgery. The findings by Subbarao *et al.* (1991) suggest that therapy should be instituted early because the pace of development and quality of speech is far superior than that of those laryngectomees whose speech therapy was delayed. However, the reasons for delay were not clearly elucidated in the paper and it is possible that some of those receiving delayed therapy had different psychosocial conditions or surgical and medical complications.

There has been research indicating that judges can discriminate between types of success in oesophageal speech. Nine listeners of 10 male oesophageal speakers judged both relative and absolute syllable stress using a nine-point scale reliably. Thus, some qualitative aspects of speech can be judged by normal untrained listeners indicating that methods are available for evaluation (Doyle *et al.*, 1989; Walker and Morris, 1988). However, the effect of listener sophistication on the judgements of tracheoesophageal intelligibility does play a role. The experienced listeners in this study did exhibit higher intelligibility scores than naive listeners. Despite these reliable measures being available, there are no studies that we could find comparing different speech and language therapy methods with qualitative speech outcomes.

Tracheoesophageal Puncture

Vocal restoration after laryngectomy may be impaired by a number of anatomic, physiological and psychological factors. Only 20–60% of patients are successful in obtaining functional oesophageal speech. Tracheoesophageal puncture (TEP) with a voice prosthesis provides successful speech for 80–90% of patients. Extrinsic factors, such as visual problems, improper occlusion of the trachea-stoma, general infirmity, and lack of motivation, may impair the use of a TE prosthesis even when fluent speech is obtained. Puncture site problems, such as salivary leakage and prosthetic extrusion, are other problems associated with TE speech failure. However, one of the most common reasons cited in the literature is the possibility that spasm or stricture of the pharyngo-oesophageal segments may prevent good speech. Myotomy has been used to overcome this problem (Blom *et al.*, 1986; McConnel, 1988; Schaefer and Johns, 1984; Welch *et al.*, 1979).

A prospective study of 14 total laryngectomy patients was undertaken to assess the predictive value of testing the TE segment using oesophageal insufflation. Two major questions were addressed by this study; whether, given time, the patients selected for myotomy, based on insufflation test results, would achieve successful speech without myotomy and whether the voice can be reliably judged at the time of fitting the valve or whether it is necessary to evaluate speech acquisition over a longer period of time. The results indicated that the insufflation test could predict speech production shortly after insertion of the valve. However, the test was less accurate predicting longer-term success as seven of the patients showed gradual speech improvement over the following months without the need for myotomy despite poor insufflation tests results. Of the 11 patients with successful TE speech at 6 months, 7 had unsuccessful speech at the time of fitting the valve (Callaway et al., 1992).

It has been suggested that radiation has an adverse effect on speech outcome. However, in a retrospective study of 357 patients, Schaefer and Johns (1984) found that treatment modality had no significant bearing on the attainment of oesophageal speech. Further investigation by Callaway et al. (1992), supported no link between radiation and speech success using a speech prosthesis.

A 2 year prospective study on primary tracheoesophageal puncture was carried out to evaluate the morbidity of the procedure and its success in restoring speech (Lauw et al., 1988). Fifty-two patients, 36 of whom suffered from carcinoma of the larynx and 16 carcinoma of the hypo-pharynx, were entered into the study. Thirty-three patients underwent total laryngectomy with primary pharyngeal closure. Fourteen patients had, in addition, pharyngectomy and reconstruction, and five patients had a pharyngolaryngo-oesophagectomy and gastric transposition. Speech was successful in 58%, 86% and 80% respectively using a tracheoesophageal puncture. This is particularly impressive given the low success rate of the more radical surgery for producing conventional oesophageal speech. Unfortunately, as with most studies, little information is given regarding the contribution of speech and language therapy input to achieving this success rate. It is unclear whether the surgery alone, or the surgery in addition to speech and language therapy were required. Although there have been few detailed studies, it would appear that good functional results with speech valves have been reported generally and the long term complications seem to be relatively few (Wetmore et al., 1985). Gleeson (1992), in a leader in the BMJ asks why this procedure is not used more widely and speculates that it may be due to surgeons' lack of interest in speech as a morbidity factor.

It is perhaps surprising that the role of the speech and language therapist in the management is not more clearly defined. In much of the literature it appears as if this is a surgical resolution to the problem, but this is contrary to practice in the United Kingdom where SLTs play an active and key role in the rehabilitation process.

Tracheoesophageal puncture represents a major advance in the vocal rehabilitation of the laryngectomee. Vocal rehabilitation by the Panje, Blom-Singer or Provox protheses is generally accepted as offering new hope to patients unable to acquire oesophageal speech. However, there is still controversy in the literature and limited evidence regarding selection of patients, the most appropriate timing of the intervention, and the most efficacious method of speech and language therapy. Most studies of this technique at the present time are descriptive and retrospective with little comparative data available. It had been expected that the use of a trachea stoma valve for surgical voice restoration would produce very much more intelligible speech because of the possibility for the natural phrasing mentioned previously. However, one study, which compared the difference in the intelligibility and general quality of tracheaoesophageal speech with and without a valve, revealed that there were no significant differences between whether the patient used a finger to occlude the air or the valve diverted the airstream, and that, if anything, the use of a valve in conversational speech produced distracting sounds which adversely affected naive listeners' judgements (Fujimoto *et al.*, 1991).

Conclusion

There are many research questions that still need to be addressed. There is no clear agreement as to what constitutes a successful outcome of treatment. There are many qualitative aspects of speech production, intelligibility and social acceptability that are encompassed in traditional speech and language therapy for laryngectomees which require more detailed investigation. Certain speech and language therapy techniques may be more successful than others and some speech and language therapists may achieve better outcomes at an earlier stage.

The psychological sequelae of laryngectomy are well described but none of the various methods of supporting, counselling and assisting have been investigated to establish either their acceptability or effectiveness in the short or long term.

Interestingly the need for speech and language therapy for laryngectomy patients has rarely been questioned as it has been in other fields. This acceptance may have militated against research into its efficacy. For example, a controversial but important question is whether speech and language therapists are the best people to be involved in the speech rehabilitation of these patients. Priest (1991) presents a paper detailing the re-education of speech following laryngectomy. Priest is not a speech and language therapist but a laryngectomee of some 14 years who feels that because he can demonstrate different techniques he has an advantage with assisting those who are learning this different mode of communication. Most speech and language therapists use laryngectomy patients who are experienced to assist with supporting and guiding their patient groups but few have questioned whether more detailed aspects of their work could be assisted by a 'professional laryngectomee'.

In summary, the physical and psychological effects of laryngectomy have been well described, as have the broad range of rehabilitation techniques that should be considered. Consideration of speech outcome prior to surgery has been shown to be important in vocal rehabilitation. Early intervention of speech rehabilitation has been established to be linked with improved speech outcomes but the various modes and types of speech and language therapy have not been tested adequately.

References

Barclay THC and Rao NN (1975). Epidemiology of laryngeal cancer. Laryngoscope 86: 2–5.

Blom ED, Singer SI and Haymaker RC (1986). A prospective study of tracheoesophageal speech. Archives of Otolaryngology: Head/Neck Surgery 112: 440–447.

Boyle P, Robertson AG, Gillis CR, Flatman GE and Scully C (1982). Epidemiology of laryngeal cancer in Scotland. Institute of the Royal College of Medical Science 10: 61–62.

Bronheim H, Strain J and Biller H (1991). Psychiatric aspects of head and neck surgery. General Hospital Psychiatry 13: 165–176.

Callaway E, Truelson JM, Wolf GT, Thomas-Kincaid L and Cannon S (1992). Predictive value of objective oesophageal insufflation testing for acquisition of tracheoesophageal speech. Laryngoscope 102: 704–708.

Cheesman AD (1983). Surgical management of the patient. In: Edels Y (Ed) Laryngectomy: Diagnosis to Rehabilitation. Beckenham: Croom Helm.

Doyle P, Swift ER and Haaf RG (1989). Effects of listener sophistication on judgements of tracheoesophageal talker intelligibility. Journal of Communication Disorders 22: 105–113.

Enderby P and Davies P (1989). Communication disorders: Planning a service to meet the needs. British Journal of Disorders of Communication 24: 301–331.

Fujimoto PA, Madison CL and Larrigan LB (1991). The effects of trachea-stoma valve on the intelligibility and quality of tracheoesophageal speech. Journal of Speech and Hearing Research 34: 33–36.

Gates GA, Ryan W, Cooper JC, Lawlis FG, Cantu E, Hayashi T, Lauder E, Welch R and Hearne E (1982). Current status of laryngectomy rehabilitation: Results of therapy. American Journal of Otolaryngology 3(1): 1–7.

Gleeson M (1992). Voice after laryngectomy. British Medical Journal. 304(4): 2–3.

Hartman DE and Scott DA (1974). Overt responses of listeners to alaryngeal speech. Laryngoscope 84(3): 410–416.

Lauw W, Wei W, Ho C and Lam K (1988). Immediate tracheoesophageal puncture for voice restoration in laryngopharyngeal resection. The American Journal of Surgery 156: 269–272.

Lehmann W and Krebs H (1991). Inter-disciplinary rehabilitation of the laryngectomee. Recent Results in Cancer Research 121: 442–449.

Levy J and Abramson A (1983). Immediate verbal communication following laryngectomy. Bulletin of the New York Academy of Medicine 59: 306–312.

Mathieson CM, Henderikus J and Scott JP (1990). Psychosocial adjustments after laryngectomy: A review of the literature. Journal of Otolaryngology 19(5): 331–336.

McConnel FMS (1988). Analysis of pressure generation of bolus transit during pharyngeal swallowing. Laryngoscope 98: 71–78.

McKenna JP, Fornataro-Clerici LM, McMenamin PG and Leonard RJ (1991). Laryngeal cancer: Diagnosis of treatment and speech rehabilitation. American Family Physician 44(1): 124–129.

Natvig K (1983a). Laryngectomy in Norway. Study number 3: Pre- and post-operative factors of significance to oesophageal speech acquisition. Journal of Otolaryngology 12(3): 322–328.

Natvig K (1983b). Laryngectomy in Norway. Study Number 1: Social personal and behavioral factors related to present mastery of the laryngectomy event. Journal of Otolaryngology 12(3): 155 -162.

Parker AJ (1993). Speech rehabilitation following laryngectomy in the United Kingdom. Third National Head and Neck Oncology Conference. Nottingham Conference (abstracts).

Perry A (1988). Surgical voice restoration following laryngectomy: The tracheoesophageal fistula technique (Singer Blom). British Journal of Disorders of Communication 23: 23–30.

Priest A (1991). The practice of speech after laryngectomy: discussion paper. Journal of the Royal Society of Medicine 84: 292–295.

Radford AJ (1993). The case for primary voice restoration. The therapist and patients viewpoint. Third National Head and Neck Oncology Conference. Nottingham Conference (abstracts).

Ranger D (1983). Extensive surgery for post cricoid carcinoma and subsequent vocal rehabilitation. In: Edels Y (Ed) Laryngectomy: Diagnosis to Rehabilitation. Beckenham: Croom Helm.

Richardson J (1981). Surgical and radiological effects upon the development of speech after total laryngectomy. American Journal of Otolaryngology 90: 294–297.

Richardson JL and Bourque L (1985). Communication after Laryngectomy. Journal of Psychosocial Oncology 3: 83–97.

Robin PE, Rockley T, Powell DJ and Reid A (1991). Survival of Cancer of the Larynx Related to Treatment. Journal of Otolaryngology 16: 193–197.

Salmon S (1979). Methods of Air Intake for Oesophageal Speech and Associated Problems. In: Keith R and Darley F (Eds) Laryngectomy Rehabilitation. San Diego, CA: College Hill Press.

Salmon S (1983). Artificial larynx speech: A viable means of alaryngeal communication. In: Edels Y (Ed) Laryngectomy Diagnoses to Rehabilitation. Beckenham: Croom Helm.

Schaefer SD and Johns DF (1984). Attaining functional oesophageal speech. Archives of Otolaryngology 108: 647–649.

Singer MI, Blom ED and Haymaker RC (1981). Voice restoration. Annals Otology, Rhinology and Laryngology 90: 498–502.

Smith R (1982). Creating alaryngeal speech. Ear Nose and Throat Journal 61: 18–27.

Stam HJ, Scott JP and Mathieson CM (1990). The Psychosocial Impact of a Laryngectomy: A Comprehensive Assessment. Unpublished Manuscript 1990 (as referred to in Mathieson et al., 1990).

Subbarao SP, Shenoy AM, Nanjundappa M and Anantha N (1991). Post laryngectomy rehabilitation: The case for planned early speech therapy. Indian Journal of Cancer 28: 218–222.

Vize C (1976). Rehabilitation of the voice after pharyngo laryngectomy and stomal repair. Cineradiography. Journal of Clinical Otolaryngology 1: 107–113.

Walker CN and Morris HL (1988). Perception of syllable stress in oesophageal speech. Journal of Communication Disorders 21: 59–73.

Welch RW, Luckman K and Ricks PM (1979). Manometry of the normal upper oesophageal sphincter and its alterations in laryngectomy. Journal of Clinical Investigation 63: 1036–1041.

Wetmore SJ, Krueger K and Blessing ML (1985). Long term results of the blom-singer speech rehabilitation procedure. Archives of Otolaryngology 111: 106–9.

Williams M (1994). Research Issues: The role of psychosocial data qualitative methodologies. Third National Head and Neck Oncology Conference. Nottingham Conference (abstracts).

Chapter 7
Learning Disability

Introduction

The condition under discussion in this section has been defined as 'a permanently reduced global capacity to learn' (Fryers, 1987). For the purposes of this chapter the term 'learning disability' and 'learning disabled' will be used, except where cited references use other terminology, e.g. mental handicap or mental retardation. People with this condition may require special care and provision or protection in employment or occupation, accommodation and social life throughout their lives.

People with learning disabilities are usually categorized as having mild, moderate, severe, or profound learning disability, which is no longer decided on IQ alone. Categorization is usually based on assessment of functional ability using developmental assessment and behavioural checklists.

The prevalence of mild mental handicap has been estimated as 30 in 1000, severe mental handicap as 3 in 1000 and profound mental handicap as 0.5 in 1000 (Fraser and Green, 1991).

There are many causes of learning disability. Damage may occur before, during or after birth and may be due to infections such as meningitis or encephalitis, injury, drugs or other toxins, metabolic disorders, brain disease, prematurity or chromosome abnormality, including the commonest, Down's Syndrome, and diseases and conditions due to prenatal factors such as hydrocephalus.

Sixty-five per cent of people with learning disability show no gross evidence of structural or biochemical abnormality and are learning disabled with 'no known cause'. Some of these are part of a pattern of inherited low intelligence and represent the lower end of the normal distribution of intelligence.

The most profoundly impaired group in this population are likely to suffer from additional impairments of vision, hearing and mobility. Assessment of the defects in this group is likely to be more complex and time consuming.

Speech and Language Therapy with Children

Speech and language therapists may be involved with people with learning disabilities from babyhood onwards. Some babies with learning disabilities may have problems with feeding and a speech and language therapist may be involved for this reason, sometimes as part of a multi-disciplinary team.

Some rationales of treatment have early intervention as an essential component or ideal aim. Some approaches involving routine general stimulation are recommended to start as early as possible in a child's life. One of these is the early intervention approach of Johansson for Down's Syndrome children. Goal behaviours, including sound making, are broken down into small components and are stimulated in a developmental sequence by the parents (Thomas, 1990).

Another approach which may be implemented in the first year of life is the introduction of vocabulary with signing and speech as a means of encouraging communication and language development in Down's Syndrome children (Le Prevost, 1983). The same author emphasizes the importance for Down's Syndrome children, of working directly on exercising oral musculature, of listening to and producing speech sounds in addition to signing and language work.

Early intervention depends on early diagnosis, and people with identifiable conditions such as Down's Syndrome may be more likely to experience early recognition and provision of services than those with a learning disability with no known cause.

Children with learning disability receive special education in special schools or in main stream schools with additional support. It is suggested that there may be emphasis in the curriculum on the encouragement of pre-intentional and intentional communication, regarding the development of feeding patterns, social interaction patterns, and of vocabulary and syntax through signing, symbols and speech.

Some packages of treatment are used widely to promote communication and language, e.g. the Makaton Vocabulary (Walker, 1973), the Derbyshire Language Scheme (Knowles and Madislover, 1982) and Living Language (Locke, 1985), and these approaches may be incorporated into the curriculum.

Recent approaches have stressed the importance of functional communication and aimed to increase and extend the range of the purposes of communication used by the child, such as expressing choices, requesting or refusing, and commenting in an everyday context. The curriculum for the child may be structured so that even the earliest reflexive and reactive responses to the environment can be recognized to perform these communicative functions (Coupe and Goldbart, 1988).

The speech and language therapist may provide input, either directly to the child, or indirectly through the devising of programmes of routines with the teacher, parent/carer or both (CSLT, 1992). Language delay in children with learning disabilities is secondary to cognitive delay and whether or not there is a discrepancy between cognitive level and linguistic level the speech and language therapist may work with the aim of enabling the child to progress to the next developmental linguistic stage.

As a child grows older there may be increasing emphasis on effective use of communication skills already present and how these are used in conversation and interactions. For example, the Social Use of Language Programme (SULP) has been devised by Rinaldi (1992) to encourage conversational skills in people with mild-to-moderate learning disability.

Speech and Language Therapy with Adults

Speech and language therapy with adults with profound handicaps aims to encourage communication behaviour of all kinds. Individualised Sensory Environments (Bunning, 1990) aims at the development of intentional communication. The client is assessed with a range of materials, stimulating particularly tactile and kinaesthetic senses. The materials most motivating to the client are then used to encourage the client to relate to objects, to people and then to objects and people together in early communication behaviour such as joint attention and requesting. There are no published evaluations of this work at present.

Joint approaches between speech and language therapists, music, art, dance and drama therapists to encourage and promote communication in the widest sense, may be used with adults (van der Gaag and Dormandy, 1993, pp. 149–150) and are particularly useful with this group of clients.

Reichle and Johnston (1993) claim that communication intervention is a crucial component of procedures used in the treatment of people showing challenging behaviour where that behaviour is found to have a communicative function. The authors stress the importance of devising a means of communication for the learner that will be as efficient as the challenging behaviour it is intended to replace.

Non-verbal communication

Since the growth in the use of alternative and augmentative systems of communication, the teaching of signs has been widely undertaken with adults as well as with children. Recent increased emphasis on the functionality of therapeutic approaches has led to concern that people in the client's environment and in the wider community should use and understand signing. Attempts have been made to find effective ways of training carers and peers to use and respond to signing (Hooper and Bowler,

1991). Symbols such as those devised by the Makaton Vocabulary Development Project (1985) have been introduced with adults as an alternative communication system, to augment existing spoken or signed communication, or to assist staff and carers to communicate with clients, e.g. by the production of such things as timetables, sets of instructions for activities and minutes of meetings in symbol form.

The emphasis on non-verbal aspects of communication in the general population has led to the development of social skills training for a number of groups of people (Argyle, 1975). People with learning disabilities have particular problems with social skills (Hitchins and Spence, 1991), and speech and language therapists have, with other professionals, engaged in teaching the extra-linguistic skills of facial expression, gesture, proximity and intonation to people with learning disabilities using a social skills approach (Argyle, 1981; Spence, 1980).

Calculator and Bedrosian (1988) stress the importance in work with adults, of considering their use of communication rather than their form of language and urge intervention designed to expand the functions of communication and promote spontaneous use, combined with providing environments that will foster the development and use of communication.

Environment

Because of the increasing awareness of the importance of the environment for the communication of people with learning disabilities, recent approaches, e.g. INTECOM (Jones, 1990), ENABLE (Hurst Brown and Keens, 1990), offer suggestions for ways to manipulate the environment in order to provide the client with the maximum opportunities for communication. Jones's approach offers training to carers in considering the client's network of relationships, daily routines and interaction with carers, to examine ways in which opportunities can be planned to extend the clients social contacts and chances to initiate communication.

ENABLE (Hurst Brown and Keens, 1990), 'encouraging a natural and better life experience', is a complete programme to encourage functional communication skills in people with learning disability. The programme is administered by a speech and language therapist trained in its use. It incorporates:

1. A training schedule for carers.
2. Assessment, intervention and resource material for:
   • the individual person with learning disabilities,
   • the group in which the individual spends most time,
   • the location (e.g. day centre) of the group.

Assessments are carried out on the individual, the group and the location, priorities assigned in parallel for all three and strategies for intervention outlined. The carer takes the main role in the intervention with some assessment and carer training being undertaken by the speech and language therapist.

Consideration of the environment of the person with learning disability has been influenced by the notion of normalization or social role valorization (Wolfensberger, 1983) which proposes the 'creation, support and defense of valued social roles for people who are at risk of devaluation'. This concept has had many influences on the work of speech and language therapists in this field, one of which has been to challenge the use of materials and techniques inappropriate for the chronological age of the person and therapists have needed to change these to incorporate suitable age-appropriate materials. This movement has raised the consciousness of workers in the field of the restricted and powerless lives experienced by many people with learning disability and complemented the emerging movements of advocacy and self-advocacy, which have had a continuing impact on the provision of services. Recently, the idea of disability in general as a problem of the individual has been challenged and it has been suggested that it is society's failure to acknowledge and meet the needs of disabled people that is responsible for many of the problems of the disabled individual (e.g. Oliver, 1992).

Efficacy of Speech and Language Therapy for Children

Bryen and Joyce (1985) undertook a critical review of 43 language intervention studies published during the 1970s. These authors found that while many of the studies aimed for the achievement of a training item during a structured session, insufficient attention was paid to the carry over of the item into everyday life. Only a third of the studies mentioned this. All of these were successful to varying degrees in terms of having some functional impact. However, more recent studies have placed central emphasis on the effect of intervention on function.

Pre-verbal communication

Warren *et al.* (1993) used a multiple baseline across subjects designed to investigate the effectiveness of facilitating the pre-linguistic skill of requesting in four developmentally delayed children, aged 23–30 months at the start of the intervention. Trainers followed the child's lead in activities with toys, asked questions and provided verbal prompts or physical assistance to enable the child to meet criteria for intentional

communication. It was found that these methods were effective in elicit-
ing the requesting behaviours of looking, or vocalization, in all the children. In addition it was found that teachers untrained in the facilitation
methods increased their interaction following intervention, which
suggests that the teachers may have been responding to the changed
behaviour of the children.

Watson and Knight (1991) describe intensive interactive teaching
with six children between the ages of 10 and 19 years with very severe
learning difficulties. Using this method, a member of staff works one-to-
one with pupils observing and responding to any movement, expression, or sound, with the aim of building a communicative relationship
and to promote initiation, eye contact, turn taking and understanding of
cause and effect. Sessions were videotaped and notes were made as
soon after the sessions as possible. The authors report that there were
noticeable improvements in such aspects as communication, social
interaction, turn taking and motor control. Staff involved believed the
treatment to be effective in building up a relationship with individual
pupils and in increasing effective observation and participation in the
classroom generally.

Comprehension

Kim and Lombardino (1991) aimed to assess the effects of 'script' context
versus 'non-script' contexts in treatment of the language comprehension
of four mentally retarded pre-school children. A script context is one
where new vocabulary or linguistic structures are presented in the
contexts of an everyday activity. A non-script context introduces vocabulary or linguistic structures during an activity with objects which is not
related to any goal. Attempts were made to teach two constructions,
'Agent Action Object', 'Action Object Locative' in two conditions, the
script context of food preparation and the non-script contexts of activities with objects. The subjects showed gains in their comprehension
under both conditions. However, the authors contend that the acquisition trends of the children indicate that the script context was the superior framework. There was a slightly better treatment effect for the Agent
Action Object construction. There is need of replication of these results
because of the small number of subjects and because using two
constructions, in addition to the script contexts, has the effect of diluting
the strength of the results.

Another approach to encouraging more effective comprehension of
language is to encourage children to request clarification if they do not
understand. Ezell and Goldstein (1991) used peer modelling to train five
children with mild-to-moderate retardation to request clarification.
Eight children who requested clarification of inadequate instructions at
pre-trial assessment were chosen as models. During training, a model sat

next to one of the subjects while experimenters gave instructions, including ones where the messages were inadequate in various ways: because of an interfering signal, an unfamiliar word, an instruction of excessive length or an unfamiliar idiomatic phrase. At each training session all types of inadequate message were included, the one type of inadequate message being trained was presented, both to the model and to the subject. Probe trials of the other inadequate messages were presented to the subject for the purpose of recording baseline and main-tenance scores. In addition, adequate messages were presented to both model and subject. In the course of training, two of the five children learned to request clarification through observation of the models alone. The other three learned to request clarification only after they were required to imitate, but went on to request clarification of different message types after further observation. All five generalized the training to unfamiliar message types and four of the five generalized the training to everyday situations. The authors suggest that requests for clarification may be a valuable social skill that could lead people with learning disabilities to take a more active role in social situations. The study indi-cates that the skills could be taught in classroom settings with the use of models.

In another study of the effectiveness of peer modelling, Goldstein and Mousetis (1990) studied the effects on receptive and expressive language learning of expressive modelling by peers. Six moderately severely retarded individuals aged 6.9–9.3 years who showed restricted use of two-word or three-word communications were the subject for this study. A language matrix for each subject was developed so that trials consisted of known and unknown objects and locations. One model and one target subject sat next to the experimenter facing a doll's house with furniture. The experimenter gave instructions, e.g. 'Put the bean on the couch' or placed an object with respect to location and asked 'What did I do?' All correct responses were reinforced. The incorrect responses of the models, but not of the subjects, were corrected. It was found that all the children acquired new two- or three-word object/location utterances following peer modelling.

Verbal expression

Yoder, Kaiser and Alpert (1991), examining the interaction between child characteristics and method of instruction in children with a wide range of developmental delay, found that both an environmental approach with some structured teaching (the Milieu approach), and an operant approach (the Communication Training Programme), were effective in bringing about improvements in language level. Forty children, aged between 2 and 7 years, but functioning in the cognitive and linguistic domains, like 1–4 year olds, were randomly assigned to one or other group and developmentally appropriate language goals were selected for each child. It was found that the more developmentally delayed children benefited most from the Milieu approach and the more able children from the communication training programme. The authors point out that this is in contrast to previous findings that more mentally delayed children benefit from a structured approach and more able children from an environmental approach, and stress that the study is an exploratory one and needs replication. They suggest that the results could be accounted for by the fact that the language goals varied for each child depending on his or her language level. The lower functioning children may have had vocabulary goals and the higher functioning children morphological and syntactic goals, which may have been more suited to a didactic style of teaching.

In a later study by the same authors (Yoder *et al.*, 1993), three mentally retarded children with a mean age of 43 months were taught nonsense words for categories of objects in two conditions. Fifteen-minute sessions were conducted for 4 days per week for a total of 64 sessions for each condition. Each child learnt the words more efficiently when they were taught 'following the child's lead', that is, when they were already showing sustained interest in the target object, than when they were taught by means of 'recruiting the child's attention', that is, when the child's attention was directed away from an object of interest and towards the target object before intervention began. The authors suggest that the study supports following the child's lead during early noun vocabulary teaching.

Tirapelle and Cipani (1992) used the 'missing item' format to develop requesting in two children, one 5 years old, one 6 years old. When the children were called to participate, in snack time in the classroom, various items necessary to carry out the activity would be missing, one at a time. During training sessions, requests for the missing item were prompted. Generalization training was undertaken so that the children responded during different activities, with different people and at different proximities to the adult. Once the requesting behaviour was established, experimenters trained the children in multiple requests by providing insufficient of the requested item and prompting responses for more. Both children responded to this training and, at the end of the treatment, were able to make appropriate requests in all the post-intervention assessments. The children varied in the number of treatment trials required to establish the behaviour. This approach offers a potentially effective way to manipulate the environment, but more work is required to establish which individual children would be helped by this technique. Although the principles of the procedure are described sufficiently to allow replication, the exact nature of the prompt given to the children during training trials in this study is not described.

Schery and O'Conner (1992) investigated the effectiveness of a school-based computer language training programme with 52 severely handicapped school children with a chronological age between 3.3 years and 12.9 years and a developmental age of at least 15 months. The children were assigned to one of two treatments phases, each of 10 weeks duration, where they received individual interactive therapy with an object matching computer programme (PEAL). Graduate students in communication disorders interacted with the child to match and explore the objects illustrated on the computer screen. The students were free to vary the content and programme levels. Analysis at the end of the treatment period indicated that the children benefited from the intervention. During the first phase of treatment the children receiving treatment showed an improvement in recognition of the vocabulary featured in the programme significantly above phase 2 subjects. During phase 2 treatment, the group 2 subjects made significant gains while phase 1 subjects stayed about the same. There was no significant difference between the groups at follow-up 6 weeks later after all training had finished when both groups had maintained the improvement in vocabulary. However, it is unclear to what extent the improvement was brought about by the computer programme itself, and to what extent by individual input from the graduate trainee, and how individual children might have differed in their response to the treatment.

Signing

Attempts have been made to assess whether signing accelerates the learning of receptive or expressive spoken language in children. There have been a number of studies comparing the introduction of language through the total communication approach using spoken words and signs, with that using words alone (Abrahamson *et al.*, 1985; Gibbs and Carswell, 1988; Jago *et al.*, 1984; Matheson, 1986; Romski and Ruder, 1984; Weller and Mahoney, 1983).

Results are equivocal, some showing no advantage of sign and speech over speech alone. Abrahamson, Cavallo and McCluer (1985) suggest that the sign advantage may be for vocabulary only and that a total communication presentation has no advantage for the development of syntax, though this may be an artefact of how signs are taught. This study found that the Down's Syndrome children in the group showed an advantage for sign, learning more quickly vocabulary presented to them with signing, but that other handicapped children did not.

Some studies of individual Down's Syndrome children have found that these children find the use of signing helpful in early vocabulary acquisition (Gibbs and Carswell, 1988; Kouri, 1989; Layton and Savino, 1990). For example, Gibbs and Carswell (1988) describe a single case study in which a 14-month-old Down's Syndrome child with oral motor problems and a hearing loss was taught a list of words under two conditions, oral and total communication. Words were matched on phonetic complexity and reinforcement value and randomly assigned to each group. After 6 months of training in play sessions four times a week, 17 words from the total communication group and four words from the oral group had been acquired.

There has been concern that signing reduces the pressure on the child to learn oral speech and thus retards oral language development, but there is no evidence from any of these studies that the use of signing slows down the acquisition of speech.

Symbols

Symbols may be used as a means of enabling the individual to communicate basic needs, acquire vocabulary or syntax or to progress towards literacy skills. In addition, many people with additional physical handicaps find symbol systems useful as an augmentative or alternative form of communication.

In a series of investigations, Rhyner (1988) studied the acquisition of language concepts using speech and non-speech systems. In the first study (cited in Rhyner 1988), 20 handicapped pre-school children participated. In the second study, the subjects were 11 Down's Syndrome children, who had been subjects in the earlier study and were thought to have performed better on the treatment tasks. These subjects were randomly assigned to one of the treatment conditions. Words were taught by means of five presentations:

1. Speech only.
2. Bliss symbols only.
3. Rebus symbols only.
4. Speech and Bliss symbols.
5. Speech and Rebus symbols.

Subjects were seen for 12 individual sessions for training in the comprehension and expression of concepts. Ten concepts were selected at random for each subject from a list of 20.

Although the author claims that the subjects taught using both speech and non-speech systems (i.e. 4, 5) needed fewer prompts to acquire the concepts, no significant treatment effects were found. Any conclusions must be tentative as there was a maximum of three children in each treatment condition.

Angelo and Goldstein (1990) describe a pragmatic teaching strategy for teaching requesting, using a communication board, for four children with mild-to-moderate developmental delay. All children had limited speech. The words chosen were: 'what', 'where' and 'who'. All children learned to point to the appropriate symbol on their board and generalized to point to the symbol during different activities in the classroom. There was no opportunity for long term follow-up to see if the skills were maintained.

Training for carers

It has been noted that parents of developmentally delayed children behave differently in conversation from those of normally developing children.

In a study by Byrne and Buchley (1993), nine Down's Syndrome children and their mothers were compared with nine normally developed children matched on TROG scores. It was found that the mothers of Down's Syndrome children had significantly shorter mean length utterance (MLU) and that the longest MLU of the Down's Syndrome children was elicited by asking questions of particular types. The authors suggest that training parents in alternative strategies of managing conversation would be useful in extending the linguistic ability of children with Down's Syndrome.

Interactive models of language intervention aim to modify the interaction style of care givers to become more responsive to the child's attempts at communication and less dominant and directive. Tannock, Girolametto and Siegel (1990) state that a number of studies have found this approach to be effective in altering parent/child interaction but that improvement in children's abilities are less consistently observed. In their evaluation of the Hanen programme, a parent focused language intervention programme espousing an interactive model, Tannock, Girolametto and Siegel (1990) assigned two groups of 16 children randomly to an experimental group, and to a control group who were treated 12 weeks later. The experimental group underwent the Hanen programme. After intervention, treatment mothers used more comments, provided specific verbal labels for objects to which the child was attending and decreased the use of specific referents, e.g. 'that one', more than control mothers. These changes were consistent with programme objectives.

The authors conclude that the programme was effective in decreasing maternal directiveness and increasing commenting and labelling in their group of highly educated and motivated parents. Despite this, they found no significant child treatment effects. The need to treat the delayed treatment control group prevented the examination of the possibility of treatment effects occurring beyond the treatment phase.

A subsequent evaluation of this study (Girolametto et al., 1993) in which participating mothers were sent questionnaires, to rate satisfaction with the programme they had received, showed that, though the parents who responded claimed their communication behaviour had changed in response to the training, video recordings of mothers, interacting with their child before and after training, showed no significant association between what the mothers reported and objective data. The authors conclude that consumer satisfaction is inadequate as a sole measure of treatment outcome.

Cullen (1988), in his review of training staff for working with mentally handicapped people, asserts that, though staff training may be received enthusiastically by participants and may increase morale in the short term, it is likely to be ineffective unless management and organizational structures are also changed.

Efficacy of Speech and Language Therapy for Adults

There are few studies of direct treatment with adults. Bryen and Joyce (1985) found that only 4.6% of the 43 studies of the efficacy of treatment published during the 1970s had, as subjects, people over the age of 22 years and this pattern has prevailed in more recent studies, most of which are of pre-school or school-age children.

We have found little recent experimental work to evaluate the efficacy of direct treatment for adults. Powell and Morrison (1994) investigated whether the use of signing by adults with learning disabilities was useful in increasing their intelligibility. Four male Down's Syndrome subjects with a mean age of 34 years were video-taped and recorded saying a series of elicited or spontaneous words and phrases under two conditions. In the 'high-signing' condition the person that the individual was interacting with used key-word signing, in the 'low-signing' condition, he or she did not. Two of the speakers were rated by the investigators as poor speakers and two as good speakers. The recordings were rated by three types of rater who did not know the subject, a trained listener who knew the signs, a skilled listener with no knowledge of signs (a Speech and Language Therapist from another speciality), and two novice listeners. All the recordings were rated in a 'seen' condition–where the rater could both see the video and hear the recording of the subjects speech–and an 'unseen' condition–where the rater could only hear the recording.

It was found that in the high-signing condition both good and poor speakers were rated as more intelligible in both seen and unseen conditions than in the low-signing condition. In the low-signing condition poor speakers were unintelligible in the unseen condition. This suggests that the use of signing may improve intelligibility of speech. The authors warn that the sample size was too small to enable meaningful significance to be shown and are attempting to repeat the study with a larger sample.

Van der Gaag and Dormandy (1993, pp. 146–147) give case descriptions of effective individual therapy with adults and suggest that such treatment can be successful if client or carer is well-motivated. However, these authors point out that some clinicians feel that such therapy is ineffective and are trying different models of service delivery. Group work and training may be considered more appropriate in this population, which is likely to have a high percentage of people with communication problems. For example, Elstob (1986) described a group approach to treatment of adults incorporating direct treatment combined with staff training.

Jones, Turner and Heard (1992) describe the model where speech and language therapists act as 'consultants and facilitators' to train staff and family in the use of total communication. The therapists collected signs, symbols and spoken words for concepts vital in the person's everyday life, which were then used together in various environments. The authors claim that social services and health service staff became increasingly willing to teach language skills as it became clear that it helped their clients and made their own lives easier.

Cameron, Lester and Lacey (1988) held a group for adults with learning difficulties aiming to facilitate the skills of interaction and initiation. Their aim was to allow clients to take the lead in modelling skills to other group members. The therapists found that they needed to monitor and change their own verbal and non-verbal behaviour in order for this to happen effectively.

Nind and Hewett (1994) advocate the technique of 'Intensive Interaction' as an appropriate way to work with adults with severe learning difficulties which can bring about developments in looking, increased time spent in interactive activity, improved ability to reciprocate warm physical contact and improved responses on communication abilities, as assessed by the Pre-Verbal Communication Schedule of Kiernan and Reed (1987).

Training for carers

The emphasis in work with adults has been on training carers and manipulating the environment to maximize the clients potential to communicate. Several staff training packages are available, e.g. ENABLE (Hurst Brown and Keen, 1990); INTECOM (Jones, 1990) but, so far, there has been little evaluation of their effectiveness.

Granlund, Terneby and Olsson (1992), used questionnaires and assessments completed by staff in an attempt to evaluate the effectiveness of a training package for staff. They found that profoundly handicapped clients experienced more opportunities for communicative interaction following a year-long structured staff-training programme, which followed a pyramidal approach–i.e. a number of staff were trained and they in turn trained other staff. Disappointingly, the communicative ability of the same adults had shown no change during that time. However, the assessment of 'communicative opportunities' were done by means of before and after rating by the care-givers who had taken part in the training, so questions about the actual effects on the environment remain unanswered.

Training communicative partners to enable the client to achieve as many communicative opportunities as possible is as important with augmentative communication as with spoken language. The use of symbol boards creates abnormal environmental grouping. Efforts are required to make social contact and the aid itself can be a distraction from the message. Even at its fastest, the method is considerably slower than speech and can be tiring.

Light (1988) reports that users of augmentative systems have few opportunities to communicate and are often pre-empted by others in their surroundings who may anticipate their needs. When people using augmentative systems interact with natural speakers, the speakers tend to dominate and initiate, and the augmentative and alternative communication systems (AAC) users tend to respond.

Light *et al.* (1992) describes a study across three dyads to train facilitators to provide more opportunities to communicate. Video-recordings showed, that following instruction, facilitators decreased their initiations and increased the proportion of their conversational turns that were responsive.

Calculator (1988) called for practitioners to adopt more functional orientations when selecting the content and evaluating the effectiveness of AAC programmes. Light (1988) points out that ratings of communicative competence of AAC users, tend to be based on patterns of 'normal' conversation that may not be appropriate for AAC.

Facilitated communication

One area where there has been recent investigation of direct work with adults is that of facilitated communication. Facilitated communication (FC) is a method where the client is physically supported by the facilitator holding the clients finger, hand, wrist, elbow or shoulder to enable the client to point to an alphabet board, or activate a typewriter, or other communication aid. It has been described in use with physically handicapped people (Crossley and Remington-Gurney, 1992), but has been used more recently with autistic people and people with learning disabilities (Biklen, 1990).

The method is highly controversial in that people thought to be severely communicatively impaired are alleged to have produced complex messages by this means. There have been a number of recently published studies that have sought to establish whether the message originated with the client or with the facilitator.

Klewe (1993) investigated 10 facilitators working with 17 people in institutions for severe mental and physical handicaps and found, in a picture-naming task, there was a relation between the picture and the answer given in almost all cases where the facilitator could see the picture. However, this relation was absent when the facilitator could not see the picture.

Szempruch and Jacobson (1993) investigated message passing in 23 severely or profoundly mentally retarded participants and their facilitators of choice and found no participant was able to accurately label or describe an object shown to them, with facilitation.

Supporters of FC object to attempts made to establish the validity of communications using a picture-naming task because of the possibility of word-finding difficulty in clients, all of whom have impairments of spoken language. Moore, Donovan and Hudson (1993) evaluated facilitated communication in five individuals, four of whom were diagnosed as intellectually impaired, in a more conversational approach suggested by their facilitators. Subjects were shown objects and talked to about topics while the facilitators were not present. The facilitators were then free to interact with the subjects as they wished in order to find out what objects had been presented and topics discussed. The facilitated output failed to yield any of the correct objects or topics even though some of the subjects used speech to name the objects correctly in their interaction with the facilitator.

Bligh and Kupperman (1993) described an evaluation of facilitated communication that had been used in a court case where the facilitated communication of a mentally retarded 7-year-old had produced accusations of abuse. Questions were put under three conditions. It was found that the facilitated output was correct only when the facilitator had both heard the question which was put to the subject and knew the answer to it. Questions unheard by the facilitator produced irrelevant output. Questions heard, where the answer was not known by the facilitator, resulted in relevant but inaccurate output.

Proponents of facilitated communication oppose quantitative evaluation of the phenomenon because they believe that such attempts break the atmosphere of trust essential for such communication to work, but investigators using quantitative methods have drawn attention to the willingness of people to take part in the studies. Early descriptions of FC, give insufficient subject or methodological details to enable evaluation or replication. It has been claimed (Crossley and Remington-Gurney, 1992) that some people needing facilitated communication at the start of the intervention became able to communicate independently after varying amounts of time, and, as Duchan (1993) suggests, there is a need for detailed qualitative studies of successful communicators. Meanwhile there is a growing body of evidence that facilitators have influenced communication. Any communication elicited in this way should be regarded with great care.

Conclusion

These studies indicate that children with learning disability can acquire new vocabulary and language structures through treatment. However, the term learning disability covers a wide spectrum of ability. Abilities have been assessed in these studies in different ways and there is a continuing problem of specifying which treatment is likely to work with which child. Whitehurst and Fishchel (1994), in their review of the outcome of early developmental language delay, found that children with secondary language impairment including mental retardation (learning disability) were at risk of later problems and assert that 'demonstrably effective early interventions . . . are badly needed . . .'.

There is an urgent need to undertake evaluations of the direct individual and group treatment that is being carried out with adults.

Attempts have been made to evaluate direct treatment, e.g. of social skills training (Millner and Dalby, 1992), by means of questionnaires but the authors have found this inadequate in identifying improvements in communication, which they and others believed to have taken place. Verification that improvement has occurred can be a problem in all branches of speech and language therapy because communication is variable and is usually assessed by means of a sample, but is particularly difficult in the area of learning disability where any improvements may be very small and subtle. There is a need for outcome measures that will identify such improvements.

Speech and language therapists working in the field of learning disabilities spend a high proportion of their time giving training and advice to carers. Recent assessments, e.g. CASP, PCP, emphasize the importance of the environment. Schemes have been developed to train staff in the manipulation or exploration of the environment in full to provide communicative opportunities, e.g. Jones (1990). A sensitive way to evaluate the effects of training and the impact of environmental approaches on the lives of clients is needed given the present emphasis by therapists.

References

Abrahamson A, Cavallo M and McCluer J (1985). Is the sign advantage a robust phenomenon? From gesture to language in two modalities. Merrill-Palmer Quarterly 31(2): 177–209

Angelo DH and Goldstein H (1990). Effects of a pragmatic teaching strategy for requesting information by communication board users. Journal of Speech and Hearing Disorders 55: 231–243.

Argyle M (1975). Bodily Communication. London: Methuen.

Argyle M (1981). Social Skills and Mental Health. London: Methuen.

Biklen D (1990). Communication unbound: Autism and praxis. Harvard Educational Review 60: 291–314.

Bligh S and Kupperman P (1993). Brief report: Facilitated communication evaluation procedure accepted in a court case. Journal of Autism and Developmental Disorders 23(3:) 553–557.

Bryen DN and Joyce DG (1985). Language intervention with the severely handicapped: A decade of research. Journal of Special Education 19(1): 7–39.

Bunning K (1990). Out of this world. Therapy Weekly. 2 August.

Byrne A and Buchley S (1993). The significance of maternal speech styles for children with Down's Syndrome. Down's Syndrome: Research and Practice 1(3): 107–117.

Calculator SN (1988). Evaluating the effectiveness of AAC programmes for persons with severe handicaps. Augmentative and Alternative Communication 4: 177–179.

Calculator SN and Bedrosian JL (1988). Communication Assessment and Intervention for Adults with Mental Retardation. London: Taylor & Francis.

Cameron L, Lester R and Lacey B (1988). Developing interaction and initiation skills in a group of adults with learning difficulties. CST Bulletin 438: 3.

Coupe J and Goldbart J (1988). Communication before speech: Normal development and impaired communication. Beckenham: Croom Helm.

Crossley R and Remington-Gurney J (1992). Getting the words out: facilitated communication training. Topics in Language Disorders 12(4): 29–45.

CSLT (1992). Communicating Quality : Professional Standards for Speech Therapists. London: The College of Speech and Language Therapy.

Cullen C (1988). A review of staff training: The Emperor's old clothes. Irish Journal of Psychology 9: 309–323.

Duchan JF (1993). Issues raised by facilitated communication for theorizing and research on autism. Journal of Speech and Hearing Research 36: 1108–1119.

Elstob L (1986). Joint implementation – An intensive approach to adult training centre problems. CST Bulletin, 416: 1–2.

Ezell HK and Goldstein H (1991). Observational learning of comprehension monitoring skills in children who exhibit mental retardation. Journal of Speech and Hearing Research 34: 141–154.

Fraser B and Green M (1991). Changing perspectives on mental handicap. In: Fraser WI, MacGillivray RC and Green AM (Eds) Hallas' Caring for People with Mental Handicaps. Oxford: Butterworth Heinemann.

Fryers T (1987). Epidemiological issues in mental retardation. Journal of Mental Deficiency Research. 31: 365–384.

Gibbs ED and Carswell LE (1988). Early use of total communication with a young Down's Syndrome child. A procedure for evaluating effectiveness. Paper presented at Council for Exceptional Children Conference, Washington DC.

Girolametto L, Tannock R and Siegel L (1993). Consumer-oriented evaluation of interactive language intervention. American Journal of Speech Language Pathology 3: 41–51.

Goldstein H and Mousetis L (1990). Effects of expressive modelling on generalized language learning by mentally retarded youth. In: Olswang LB, Thompson CK, Warren SF and Minghetti NJ (Eds) Treatment Efficacy Research in Communication Disorders. Rockville, MD: American Speech-Language-Hearing Foundation.

Granlund M, Terneby J and Olsson C (1992). Creating communicative opportunities through a combined in-service training and supervision package. European Journal of Special Needs Education 7(3): 229–252.

Hitchins A and Spence R (1991). The Personal Communication Plan (PCP). Windsor: NFER-Nelson.

Hooper H and Bowler DM (1988). Peer tutorship of manual signs by mentally retarded adults. Summary of dissertation submitted in partial fulfilment of MSc.

Hurst Brown L and Keens A (1990). ENABLE: Encouraging a natural and better life experience. London: Forum Consultancy.

Jago JL, Jago AG and Hart M (1984). An evaluation of the total communication approach for teaching language skills to developmentally delayed preschool children. Education and Training of the Mentally Retarded 19(3): 175–182.

Jones J (1990). INTECOM: A Package Designed to Integrate Carers into Assessing and Developing the Skills of People with Learning Difficulties. Windsor: NFER-Nelson.

Jones J, Turner J and Heard A (1992). Making communication a priority. CSLT Bulletin 478: 6–7.

Kiernan C and Reed B (1987). Pre-Verbal Communication Schedule. Windsor: NFER-Nelson.

Kim YT and Lombardino LJ (1991). The efficacy of script contexts in language comprehension intervention with children who have mental retardation. Journal of Speech and Hearing Research 34: 845–857.

Klewe L (1993). Brief report: An empirical evaluation of spelling boards as a means of communication for the multihandicapped. Journal of Autism and Developmental Disorders 23(3): 559–566.

Knowles W and Madislover M (1982). The Derbyshire Language Scheme. Ripley: Derbyshire County Council Education Department.

Kouri T (1989). How manual sign acquisition relates to the development of spoken language: A case study. Speech and Hearing Services in Schools 20: 50–62.

Layton TL and Savino MA (1990). Acquiring a communication system by speech and sign in a child with Down's Syndrome; A longitudinal investigation. Child Language, Teaching and Therapy 6(1): 59–76.

Le Prevost P (1983). Using the Makaton vocabulary in early language training with a Down's baby: A single case study. Mental Handicap 11(2): 28–29.

Light J (1988). Interaction involving individuals using augmentative and alternative communication systems: State of the art and future directions. Augmentative and Alternative Communication 4(2): 66–82.

Light J, Dattilo J, English J, Gutierrez and Hartz J (1992). Instructing facilitators to support the communication of people who use augmentative communication systems. Journal of Speech and Hearing Research 35: 865–875.

Locke A (1985). Living Language. Windsor: NFER-Nelson.

Makaton Vocabulary Development Project (1985). Symbols for Makaton. MVDP. Camberley.

Matheson PB (1986). Evaluation of a total communication approach for pre-school aged children with Down's Syndrome. PhD thesis, Hosstra University.

Millner L and Dalby M (1992). An evaluation of an assertiveness course offered to people with a mild or moderate mental handicap. Mental Handicap 20: 21–26.

Moore S, Donovan B and Hudson A (1993). Brief report: Facilitator-suggested conversational evaluation of facilitated communication. Journal of Autism and Developmental Disorders 23(3): 541–552.

Nind M and Hewett D (1994). Access to Communication. London: David Fulton.

Oliver M (1992). Changing the social relations of research production? Disability, Handicap and Society 7(2): 101–114.

Powell G and Morrison C (1994). Human Communication May–June 3(3): 16–18.

Reichle J and Johnston SS (1993). Replacing challenging behaviour: The role of communication intervention. Topics in Language Disorders 13(3): 61–67.

Rhyner PM (1988). Graphic symbol and speech training of young children with Down's Syndrome: Some preliminary findings. Journal Of Childhood Communication Disorders 12(1): 25–47.

Rinaldi W (1992). The Social Use of Language Programme. Windsor: NFER-Nelson.

Romski MA and Ruder KF (1984). Effects of speech and speech and sign instruction on oral language learning and generalization of action plus object combinations by

Down's Syndrome children. Journal of Speech and Hearing Disorders 49: 293–302.

Schery TK and O'Conner LC (1992). The effectiveness of school-based computer language intervention with severely handicapped children. Language Speech and Hearing Services in Schools 23: 43–47.

Spence S (1980). Social Skills Training with Children and Adolescents. Windsor: NFER-Nelson.

Szempruch J and Jacobson JW (1993). Evaluating facilitated communications of people with developmental disabilities. Research in Developmental Disabilities 14: 253–264.

Tannock R, Girolametto L and Siegel L (1990). Are the social-communicative and linguistic skills of developmentally delayed children enhanced by a conversational model of language intervention? In: Olswang LB, Thompsom CK, Warren SF and Minghetti NG (Eds) Treatment Efficacy Research in Communication Disorders. Rockville, MD: American Speech Language and Hearing Foundation.

Thomas E (1990). Early intervention in Down's Syndrome. Speech Therapy in Practice May: 4–5.

Tirapelle L and Cipani E (1992). Developing functional requesting: Acquisition, durability and generalization of effects. Exceptional Children 58(3): 260–269.

van der Gaag A and Dormandy K (1993). Communication and Adults with Learning Disabilities. London: Whurr.

Walker (1973). An experimental evaluation of the success of a system of communication for the deaf mentally handicapped (1978). Unpublished Master's Thesis, University of London.

Warren SF, Yoder PJ, Gazdag GE, Kim K and Jones HA (1993). Facilitating prelinguistic communication skills in young children with developmental delay. Journal of Speech and Hearing Research 36: 83–97.

Watson J and Knight C (1991). An evaluation of intensive interactive teaching with pupils with very severe learning difficulties. Child Language Teaching and Therapy 7(3): 310–325.

Weller EL and Mahoney GJ (1983). Comparison of oral and total communication modalities on the language training of young mentally handicapped children. Education and Training of the Mentally Retarded 18(2): 103–110.

Whitehurst GJ and Fishchel E (1994). Practitioners review: Early developmental language delay. What, if anything, should the clinician do about it? Journal of Child Psychology and Psychiatry 34(4): 613–648.

Wolfensberger W (1983). Social role valorisation: A proposed new term for the principle of normalisation. Mental Retardation 21: 234–239.

Yoder PJ, Kaiser AP and Alpert CL (1991). An exploratory study of the interaction between language teaching methods and child characteristics. Journal of Speech and Hearing Research 34: 155–167.

Yoder PJ, Kaiser AP, Alpert C and Fischer R (1993). Following the child's lead when teaching nouns to preschoolers with mental retardation. Journal of Speech and Hearing Research 36: 158–167.

Chapter 8
Part One: Stammering

Introduction

Stammering[1] is characterized by stoppages and disruptions in fluency that interrupt the flow of speech. These stoppages may take the form of repetitions of sounds, syllables or words, or may be due to the prolongation of sounds and can involve silent blocking of the airflow for speech. Persons who stammer have difficulty in controlling their speech flow and demonstrate highly individual variability in fluency, which can relate to mood, situations, fatigue and various other individual factors.

These people are usually very aware of their difficulty, embarrassed by it, and find speaking takes extra physical and mental effort. This effort to speak will frequently result in concomitant physical movements or facial grimaces.

In addition to these overt disruptions of speech, stammerers will frequently avoid using certain words, or sounds that they predict will cause them difficulty. In this way, some dysfluency can be masked. Furthermore, a stammerer may avoid talking in some situations or to some people. Many authors also attribute certain psychological and emotional traits that may cause some element of dysfluency or be an effect of it. There is no evidence to indicate that the stammerers are any more or less intelligent, or nervous than the general population (Bloodstein, 1987), although some studies show a higher incidence of stammering associated with certain characteristics and syndromes.

Prevalence

Bloodstein (1987), discussing the problems of estimating the prevalence of stammering, summarizes the results of 38 studies of schoolchildren in the United States of America, Europe, Africa, Australia and the West

---

[1] The term 'stammer' is commonly used within the UK whilst the same condition is termed 'stutter' in the USA and some European countries. In this review the terms are used interchangeably guided by the usage in the paper under discussion.

Indies. These studies show that the prevalence of stammering is about 1%.

Andrews *et al.* (1983) came to the same conclusion; about 1% of schoolchildren, worldwide, can be considered stutterers. There are few studies of the prevalence of stuttering in very young children, or in adults, but there is some indication that stuttering declines slightly after puberty and therefore the adult rate is likely to be less than 1%.

Estimates of incidence vary between 5% and 15%. The latter figure suggested by Bloodstein (1987) includes those children who stutter only for a brief period, but these may well be children who are exhibiting normal non-fluency rather than primary stuttering. Andrews *et al.* (1983), report that the incidence appears to be about 5% when considering those who have stuttered for longer than 6 months.

Along with most other developmental speech and language disorders, stammering has a higher incidence and prevalence in boys. Studies suggest a ratio of between 3:1 to 5:1.

Causes of Stammering

There has been considerable research and even more speculation regarding the causes of stammering. Three themes have been addressed throughout the literature:

* the role of genetics and neurophysiology,
* learning theories, e.g. the role of the environment and linguistic opportunity,
* the emotional/psychological dimension.

There is substantial evidence that, as a group, stammerers differ from non-stammerers on cognitive, linguistic and motor tasks. A high proportion of stammerers show a poorer performance on central auditory processing tasks and discrimination of temporal information. Furthermore, there is a higher incidence of stammering in children who have other speech and language difficulties (Smith, 1990).

Despite this, it must be remembered that there are many stammerers who do not have these difficulties and, in addition, there are many people who speak fluently who have difficulties similar to stammerers. It is possible, therefore, that the neurophysiological difficulties may predispose the individual to stammering only if other conditions, emotional or in the environment, are realized (Peters and Guitar, 1991).

Stammering may run in families. Support for this is gained from studies of twins, families, separation, and genetic linkage. These are summarized in a paper reviewing evidence for genetic factors in stuttering (Pauls, 1990). The author concludes that whilst there is some suggested evidence of familial linkage, most studies are flawed and the evidence is, perhaps, less conclusive than was previously thought to be the case. There is a need to carry out more stringent studies to identify the role of genetics in stammering. It is still unclear as to whether there is a higher relationship within families because of genetics, imitation of speech styles, or anxious responses by dysfluent parents, exacerbating normal dysfluency (Yairi, 1993).

Many neurophysiological theories have been proposed to account for various speech difficulties (Rosenfield and Nudelman, 1987). Geschwind and Galaburda (1985) propose that the normal left hemisphere growth is delayed during fetal development, which causes speech and language functions to be localized inappropriately. Kent (1983) and Van Riper (1982) hypothesize that the disturbance of stuttering is the product of mis-timing in the pattern of neuro-muscular commands for speech, whilst Neilson and Neilson (1987) suggest that stuttering results from inadequate neuronal resources to make the necessary sensory to motor transformations for fluent speech. Peters and Guitar (1991) try to integrate all these suggestions by describing three possibilities related to speech and language processes. The processes:

1. become established in the left hemisphere structures that have reduced capacity because of slow development;
2. migrate to right hemisphere structures where temporal patterning is slower;
3. are divided between right and left hemispheres thus creating a time delay in processing.

Most authorities agree there are likely to be subgroups with different individual or causal factors.

Therapy for Stammering

Different forms of treatment to 'cure' stammering have been documented over many centuries. Potions and medications produced by herbalists, pebbles in the mouth, punishments and exorcism, were described in the Middle Ages as being efficacious. To this day, there are many different approaches to the treatment of stammering that depend upon the clinician's beliefs about the underlying nature of the stammering disorder and the ultimate goals that the client and therapist see as important. Several of the advocates for these approaches make unsubstantiated claims of the benefits whilst others refer to the methods of 'charlatans' and suggest any value can only be temporary.

There are approaches that emphasize increasing the amount of fluency and there are treatment procedures that aim to modify the stammering behaviour. The different emphases lead to different strategies during the therapy programme. Some therapy programmes depend more on monitoring and shaping the speech or articulatory behaviour and others have a psychosocial or psychoemotional basis. There are proponents of different approaches who have strong convictions regarding their own methods (Levy, 1987). The literature and conference reports indicate that there are substantial cultural differences affecting stammering therapy.

It is important to acknowledge at this stage that the literature regarding stammering, its treatment and evaluation is dominated by the USA. There are several research institutes in America dedicated to this area. But specialist therapists in the United Kingdom tend to be less behavioural in their approach and claim to tailor the therapy to the needs of individual patients rather than follow therapy programmes. It is unsurprising then that reviews of stuttering treatment (Bloodstein, 1987; Curlee and Perkins, 1969) show that behaviour-modification therapy procedures underlie many of the practices that clinicians use. There appears to be a strange dichotomy: some therapy may be seen as diffuse and eclectic in comparison with the single-minded, very specific approaches that can be taken by other clinicians. As it is likely that stammering has more than one basis and different presentations and associated problems, one could deduce that there should be more than one treatment approach; this is not reflected strongly in the literature. Complete packages of therapy are advocated for stammerers, but therapists with more general skills may select different components of these packages without necessarily conforming to their theoretical principles.

The Efficacy of Treatment

One of the difficulties in reviewing the efficacy of stammering therapy is the lack of agreement of what is a good therapeutic outcome. The definition of success of treatment is an important variable in determining the effectiveness of stuttering therapy (St Louis and Westbrook, 1987; Starkweather, 1993). Different methods of measuring speech fluency, speaking rate, attitudes; debates regarding the environments for assessments (e.g. clinic based or home based), or the time at which outcome should be measured (e.g immediately after treatment, 1–2 years later), may lead to many different approaches to evaluation in this area. Ingham (1990), who draws attention to these issues, also adds that just because 'stutterers might achieve stutter-free and even perceptually normal speech, does not mean that their speech is also acoustically, physiologically and experientially, normal.'

There is an urgent need for empirical studies to establish standard methods for determining the duration, frequency and circumstances in which a stutterer's speech should be sampled. It is also necessary to determine which aspects of the speech and psychosocial variables need to be analysed in order to reflect this disorder in its totality and thus move towards a common approach to studying the efficacy of speech therapy treatment for stammering.

Many therapists lack confidence in treating stammering and there is a general feeling that the condition is poorly understood and difficult to treat. This is at variance with the literature, which is filled with treatise on the causes, nature and effects of stammering. Whilst there is less literature on the efficacy of speech therapy treatment for stammering, it is still a convincing pool of information. But again, caution is required and we draw attention to the predominance of American research which may not necessarily allow generalization to other countries.

Most therapy programmes now contain elements of teaching the stutterer to modify the moments of stuttering as well as reducing the fear of stuttering and eliminating avoidance behaviours associated with those fears. Additionally, many therapists include work to improve stammerers attitudes to their dysfluency. Within this, there are different schools of thought which emphasize different aspects of the intervention and which advocate different ways of achieving its goals. However, all the reported studies indicate that stammering behaviour does decrease following treatment.

Overview of Studies

Reviewers of efficacy studies relating to stammering are faced with difficulties similar to therapy research with other client groups. Different researchers investigate different approaches to treatment, from the point of view of both therapy content and mode of delivery, for example, intensive, group, individual and follow-up studies. Approaches to assessments and outcome measures along with views of 'improvement', are varied and complex and in most studies make compilation difficult. Therapy programmes such as 'fluency shaping' 'prolonged speech', 'behaviourial approach' and 'smooth speech' may not be described in sufficient detail to encourage confidence that there are shared conceptual principles. Some authors use similar but distinct therapy approach terms interchangeably.

Howie, Tanner and Andrews in 1981, evaluated a 3 week programme of intensive therapy including prolongation techniques immediately after treatment and 1 year later. Thirty-six subjects were included and measures of speech and attitude were taken. At the end of the programme, all subjects showed 'near normal' fluency, but there was some deterioration in 40% of the clients 1 year later. The authors suggest that this gives them the confidence to assure clients that they have a 70% chance of having substantially improved speech and increased speaking confidence 12 months after receiving their treatment. They add that the chances of achieving normal fluency are somewhat lower, although clients can probably increase the odds by continuing speech practice.

A number of studies have examined the Van Riper approach to stammering, which includes block modification, addressing feelings and attitudes, and reducing speech pressure by emphasizing 'stutter more fluently' with planned maintenance procedures. Two carefully designed studies are now described to represent these. The first, by Metz, Samar and Sacco (1983), examined 14 patients who had received both group and individual therapy daily for 5 weeks. They noticed a dramatic decrease in stuttering behaviour and, using acoustic measurements, they were able to confirm reports in previous studies that stuttering therapy alters the acoustic properties of a stutterer's fluent speech at the same time as reducing stuttering frequency.

This replicated the study by Metz, Onufrak and Ogburn (1979), which examined nine stutterers who had three phases to their treatment:

1. To improve stuttering awareness.
2. To modify the stutter using slow onset and reduction of rate.
3. To address generalization.

Therapy for all the subjects changed the acoustic measures and the mean number of stutters was greatly reduced.

There are inherent difficulties in interpreting the results of these studies that compare fluent speech characteristics of stutterers and non-stutterers. The majority of the studies reviewed by Armson and Kalinowski (1994) have reported stutterer/non-stutterer differences in temporal parameters of fluent speech production. Such differences have been interpreted as indicating that stutterers possess temporal-motor deficits that are ever present in speech. However, a problem for researchers studying the fluent speech of stutterers, is that the samples may be contaminated by the influence of stuttering and it is likely that fluent speech of stutterers changes as a function of a number of variables.

Two studies, examining the therapeutic approach of the regulated breathing method, including awareness training, have been conducted by Waterloo and Gotestam (1988) and Ladouceur, Caron and Caron (1989). The first study looked at 32 subjects who were randomly assigned to treatment or no treatment. The treatment was extremely brief, i.e. one 3 hour session. Despite this, the authors report a marked reduction in stammering behaviour for those who were treated, both immediately following therapy and at an 8 month follow-up assessment. Results established that the stammering behaviour was less than the control group and less than the subjects pre-treatment evaluation.

The second study (Ladouceur et al., 1989) took a different approach to the evaluation of the technique. Examining nine patients on three single case multiple baseline techniques. They found that mild and moderate stammerers showed clinical improvement on fluency, behavioural and cognitive measures. None of the severe stammerers achieved clinical improvement. There have been few other studies looking at the differential improvement according to the severity of the stammer. They also found that patients self-prediction was quite accurate in predicting actual outcome. This work followed the previous study by Ladouceur and Saint Laurent (1986) where, using the same therapy programme, they compared eight stutterers receiving this treatment with eight non-stutterers. The stutterers were matched with their controls. The treatment consisted of eight 2 hour sessions of regulated breathing and awareness training. They examined and compared the amount of fluency and speed of speech in telephone conversation and public speaking. The treatment showed a decrease in stuttering, but there was no change in the rate of speech. They found that self-efficacy and prediction improved. The authors report that stammering was eliminated in the majority of subjects and that this was maintained over 6 months. It is interesting to note that they had identified that the rate of speech was different to normal subjects. This raises the issue that some stammerers whilst reducing their stammering may still not have normal speech.

This issue was addressed by Runyan, Bell and Prosek (1990) who investigated the naturalness of treated stutterers' speech. The stutterers they examined had all received different types of treatment, but they concluded that some stutterers' fluent speech is still 'un-natural' whilst other stutterer's speech can improve to a similar level of naturalness as that of normals. The treated stutterers' fluent speech was different after treatment from the fluent speech of non-stutterers, but the naturalness was not related to severity of dysfluency.

Franken *et al.* (1992) evaluating a fluency shaping (smooth speech) treatment approach with 32 severe stammerers, over a 4 week intensive course, found that the nature of outcome changed according to the time of assessment so that at pre-treatment, immediately after treatment, and at a 6 month follow up there were detectable differences between stammerers and non-stammers. Pre-therapy, the major difference was the large proportions of dysfluency. However post-therapy, there were low scores for the stammerers on both dynamics and prosody, which was probably related to the flattening effect of smooth speech treatment. Six months later, the follow up showed that the dynamics and prosody were still different from that of normals and there was a slightly increased number of dysfluencies compared with the immediate post-treatment level. Thus, therapy had affected these severe stammerers and the effects were reflected in different types of speech compared with normals both immediately following treatment and 6 months later.

Similarly, Onslow *et al.* (1992), comparing seven stutterers treated residentially for 14 days using a prolonged speech method matched with seven non-stutterers, showed changes in naturalness scores that became more disparate from normal immediately post-treatment but then improved on naturalness several weeks subsequent to the establishment of stutter-free speech.

Some therapists and researchers focus on the modification of the stammering behaviour, with no attempt to change the stammerer's attitudes, believing that the attitude will change as a consequence of behaviour change. Another school focuses the therapy programme on both attitudinal modification and behaviour change (Stewart, 1992).

There has been particular interest in the United Kingdom in the use of personal construct therapy to assist in the treatment of stammering. Faye Fransella (1972) pioneered the approach, arguing that 'the path from stuttering to fluency is a process of reconstruction'. She proposed that individuals who stutter usually construe themselves as stutterers whenever they are in verbal communication with other adults and that they have to change their perceptions to become fluent people, as well as fluent speakers.

Fransella reported her work with 20 stutterers, showing that stuttering decreased after a programme of personal construct therapy and that there was a relatively low relapse rate. However, it was noted that it took many months to achieve the results; this may have been because no specific manipulation of the speech itself was included in the research design and no treatment was given on anything other than an individual basis. Evesham and Fransella (1985), reporting a modification of this approach, evaluated the effectiveness of 48 subjects randomly assigned to a group who had treatment to improve fluency through behaviour modification with a group who had both this and additionally, personal construct therapy. All the work was done in groups, with a 2 week residential course followed by ten 1 week sessions. The authors note that there was a difference despite random allocation in the severity of stammerers between the two groups. However, both groups improved significantly on fluency and the group that experienced the additional construct therapy had a significantly lower relapse rate than those who received the speech technique alone.

The difficulties with relapse have been addressed in several papers (Starkweather, 1993). It has been noticed over several decades that many patients do well immediately after therapy, but may have difficulty in maintaining the new level of fluency.

Craig and Andrews (1985) and Andrews and Craig (1988) report a series of studies investigating the features that may predict those who will have relapses following intensive group therapy for stammering. They found the predictors of outcome were: skill mastery, i.e. the ability to control the stammer by the end of treatment; internalization of the locus of control; and normal attitudes to communication. Locus of control has been defined as 'the extent to which a person perceives events as being a consequence of his or her own behaviour' and, therefore, potentially under personal control (Lefcourt, 1976). Of those who achieved all of these by the end of therapy, 97% maintained improvement 10 months later. However, no subject who failed on one of these was able to maintain fluency at a similarly high level.

In another study by these authors (Andrews and Craig, 1988), six subjects who had unfavourable scores on one of the three measures of skill (mastery, internalization and attitudes to communication) were re-treated emphasizing locus of control. Of the six subjects, five improved their scores in this area and this led to a more favourable outcome ten months later.

Craig and Calver (1991) conducted several studies into the maintenance of fluency following treatment. The first study showed that virtually all those treated were satisfied with their fluency following treatment but this satisfaction decreased to under half in the long term (12–18 months later). The second study showed considerable opportunity in the long term for job promotion and upgrade in occupation for persons successfully completing a smooth speech programme.

The third study compared employer perceptions of their employees' speech between a group who had received treatment for stuttering and a no-treatment group. Employers' perceptions of the treatment group were significantly enhanced, whereas no significant change occurred in employers' perceptions of the control group. Of those who relapsed, the majority believed that their relapses were not due to embarrassment but to feelings that they should speak faster.

How long to continue therapy is a question that has not been answered. However, Garvin-Cullen (1990) looked at the improvement in outcomes of 50 subjects who were allocated to either a self-maintenance group or a supervised maintenance group. They found that at 6 months post-treatment, those who had had supervision in their maintenance maintained a better level of fluency and adjustment.

Boberg, Howie and Woods (1979), in a review of studies concerned with the maintenance of fluency, attempted to abstract and discuss present issues in fluency maintenance and present 'speculative positions on relapse in the hope that it will provoke further discussion and research'. The authors drew attention to the substantial progress that has been made in the establishment of fluency and the transfer of fluency. They argued that greater attention should be given to the maintenance phase so that relapse is prevented in a greater number of stammerers. The methods of supporting clients, following the termination of regular therapy, fall under the following categories:

1. Regular clinical contact following treatment.
2. Greater emphasis on self-responsibility.
3. Emphasis on the need for changing attitudes to speech, self-concepts.
4. Intensive refresher programmes or re-cycling through the initial programme.

In summary, the authors concluded that there was evidence that suggested that virtually all forms of intensive behaviourial treatment of stuttering produce immediate dramatic increases in fluency, but encounter serious relapse problems in the post-treatment environment:

> 'Maintenance remains the last and possibly the most challenging aspect of fluency management. At present a wide spectrum of maintenance strategies needs to be studied in terms of their effectiveness as therapeutic tools and also at the level of the power of the theoretical rationale on which their use is based.'

Relapse may be related to the physiological basis of the dysfluency or the fact that dysfluency may have secondary gains. Dalton (1987) argued that improvements can be maintained as long as an active programme integrating behaviourial and psychological procedure is followed.

There have been many reports of different types of approaches to stammering therapy, some of them rather novel. One consistent theme has been the debate between punishing the stammerer as compared to re-enforcing and encouraging fluency. A review of this literature by Nittrouer and Cheney (1984) concluded that the body of experimental literature indicates that operant techniques can effectively reduce stuttering, with punishment of dysfluencies producing more noticeable results than re-enforcement of fluent responses. They conclude that operant conditioning is an effective means of modifying stuttering behaviour and should be more prominent among the procedures used by speech and language therapists. However, very few treatment programmes include the theories related to punishment, whether by verbal reprimand or time-out. These approaches seem to be in direct opposition, both practically and theoretically, to the point of view that is generally taken.

Burgraff (1974) investigated the effect of a speech technique in comparison with desensitization to anxious situations in 18 subjects. The subjects all received relaxation therapy and then were randomly assigned to one of two groups. The experimental group had speech treatment for 3–4 weeks. The dysfluencies reduced by 35–40% in both groups and there was no significant difference in outcome. Surprisingly, there appeared to be no correspondence between the anxiety levels pre- and post-treatment and the severity of the stammer.

This review would be incomplete if the trials investigating the effects of neuropharmacological agents on stuttering were not, even if only briefly, mentioned. An overview of this area by Ludlow and Braun (1993) identified the design difficulties of many of the published 22 papers evaluating the effects of drugs on stammering. Whilst most of the studies were random controlled trials using double blind methods, the outcome measures were weak. The authors call for more multidisciplinary approach to trials of these kind. The two following studies illustrate the strengths and weaknesses that Ludlow and Braun have highlighted and are of note in this review. The first by Kampman and Brady (1993), investigated the effect of Bethanechol on 10 patients in a cross-over double blind trial. No significant difference between the drug and the placebo was found at the end of the study. However, two patients did find it useful and they elected to continue taking the drug for 6 months. It was postulated by the authors that some patients have a more neuro-physiological basis to their stammer and may be Bethanechol responders.

In a trial of Carbemazepine (Harvey *et al.*, 1992), patients were allocated to receiving either 400mg or 800mg of the drug. No objective improvement was found after treatment, but subjective ratings were noted with subjects reporting decreased anxiety regarding stammering.

Conclusion

It appears from this review of the literature that therapy for stammering is effective, particularly in the short term. Most stammerers will make gains and will be able to maintain fluency for some time. Techniques that combine teaching patients a strategy for overcoming their speech problem, along with psychological intervention and therapy aimed at improving attitudes, appear to be the most effective. Maintenance of improvement is a problem with approximately 50% of stammerers, but relapses frequently occur quite late on, for example after 12 months. Therapists are now investigating methods of reducing the relapse rate. Blood (1993) urges against complacency indicating the necessity to improve the methods and standards of research in this field.

Andrews, Guitar and Howie (1980), in a review of literature, found 42 studies covering treatment of a total of 756 stutterers. In order to amalgamate the results and synthesize the view on efficacy, they conducted a meta-analysis on the data available. Meta-analysis allows the integration of diverse research through statistical analysis of the results of individual studies. The dependent variable is the magnitude of treatment effect or effect size (ES), and it is calculated from the difference between treated and control group mean scores, standardized by the variability of the control group scores (Smith and Glass, 1977).

Six common principal treatment models were identified and ranked in order of effectiveness:prolonged speech, gentle onset, rhythm, airflow, attitude therapies, and systematic desensitization.

In this review, the treatment effects from 116 pre- and post-treatment pairs of measures were deduced and Andrews, Guitar and Howie (1980) concluded that stuttering treatments can be beneficial and the benefits appear comparable to other treatments in health sciences. At that time they felt that prolonged speech and gentle onset techniques showed better outcome than airflow and attitude treatment. However, all these approaches are preferable to no treatment. There have been a considerable number of extra reports that have compared and contrasted different treatment methods. Thirty efficacy studies published since 1980 and reviewed by St Louis and Westbrook (1987), strengthen Andrews *et al.*'s findings and support their conclusion that 'evidence suggests beneficial results from the treatment of stammering. Relapse over time is slow, certainly slower than with some other treatments for chronic conditions'.

But there are many questions that remain unanswered; amongst these are:

1. Is there a spectrum of stammering disorders, with those who have more biological and those who have more psychological underlying causes and are there ways of identifying these?
2. Is there a better way of classifying/categorizing stammering and stammerers?
3. What are the most appropriate things to measure to determine outcome of treatment?
4. What is the most appropriate way of supporting long-term stammerers to assist with maintenance of their fluency?
5. What lengths of treatment are required for maximum gain?
6. What skills do therapists require to treat stammerers appropriately?

Stammering has attracted an extensive amount of well-designed and challenging research compared with many other fields in speech and language therapy.

Therapists and researchers, along with patients, strive for different goals in therapy and assess different variables in different ways. This makes it difficult to be conclusive about the effectiveness, as one person's excellent result may be another's marginal failure. As with all other reviews one is struck by methodological difficulties in the field and the lack of rigour in some studies and the difficulty of pooling results. However, we can take comfort that in this area there has been increasingly vigorous long term effort to develop hypotheses and treatments and evaluate these treatments and, whilst we must not accept simplistic evaluations of clinical effectiveness, the field shows increasing sophistication in tackling these challenging issues.

References

Andrews G and Craig A (1988). Prediction of outcome after treatment for stuttering. British Journal of Psychiatry 153: 236–240.

Andrews G, Guitar B and Howie P (1980). Meta-analysis of the effects of stuttering treatment. Journal of Speech and Hearing Disorders 45: 287–307.

Andrews G, Craig A, Feyer A, Hoddinott S, Howie P and Neilson M (1983). Stuttering, a review of research findings and theories, circa 1982. Journal of Speech and Hearing Disorders 48: 226–246.

Armson J and Kalinowski J (1994). Interpreting results of fluent speech paradigm in stuttering research: Difficulties in separating cause from effect. Journal of Speech and Hearing Research 37: 69–82.

Blood G (1993). Treatment efficacy in adults who stutter: Review and recommendations. Journal of Fluency Disorders 18: 303–318.

Bloodstein O (1987). A Handbook on Stuttering. Chicago: National Easter Seal Society.

Boberg E, Howie P and Woods L (1979). Maintenance of fluency: A review. Journal of Fluency Disorders 4: 93–116.

Burgraff RI (1974). The efficacy of systematic desensitisation via imagery as a therapeutic technique with stutterers. British Journal of Disorders of Communication 9: 134–139.

Craig A and Andrews G (1985). The prediction and prevention of relapse in stuttering. Journal of Behaviour Modification 9(4): 427–442.

Craig A and Calver P (1991). Following up on treated stutterers: Studies of perceptions of fluency and job status. Journal of Speech and Hearing Research 34: 279–284.

Curlee R and Perkins W (1969). Conversational rate control therapy for stuttering. Journal of Speech and Hearing Disorders 34: 245–250.

Dalton P (1987). Maintenance of change: Towards the integration of behavioral and psychological procedures. In: P Dalton (Ed) Approaches to the Treatment of Stuttering. Beckenham: Croom Helm.

Evesham M and Fransella F (1985). Stuttering relapse: the effect of a combined speech and psychological reconstruction programme. British Journal of Disorders of Communication 20(3): 237–248.

Franken MC, Boves L, Peters H and Webster R (1992). Perceptual evaluation of speech before and after fluency shaping stuttering therapy. Journal of Fluency Disorders 17: 223–241.

Fransella F (1972). Personal Change and Reconstruction: Research on a Treatment of Stuttering. London: Academic.

Garvin-Cullen AJ (1990). The relationship between locus of control and the effectiveness of post remediation activities on the maintenance of fluency following short-term intensive behavioral therapy for stuttering. PhD Thesis Health Science, New York University.

Geschwind N and Galaburda AM (1985). Cerebral lateralisation: Biological mechanisms, associations and pathology: 1. A hypothesis and a programme for research. Archives of Neurology 42: 429–459.

Harvey JE, Culatta R, Halikas J, Sorenson J, Luxenberg M and Pearson V (1992). The effects of carbamazepine on stuttering. The Journal of Nervous and Mental Disease 180(7): 451–457.

Howie PM, Tanner S and Andrews G (1981). Short and long term outcome in an intensive treatment programme for adult stutterers. Journal of Speech and Hearing Disorders 46: 104–109.

Ingham RJ (1990). Research on stuttering treatment for adults and adolescents: A perspective on how to overcome a malaise. In: Cooper J (Ed) Research Needs in Stuttering. Roadblocks and Future Directions. Rockville, MD: ASHA Report No. 18: 91–95.

Kampman K and Brady JP (1993). Bethanechol in the treatment of stuttering. Journal of Clinical Psychopharmacology 13(4): 284–285.

Kent RD (1983). Facts about stuttering: Neuropsychologic perspectives. Journal of Speech and Hearing Disorders 48: 249–255.

Ladouceur R and Saint Laurent L (1986). Stuttering: a multi-dimensional treatment and evaluation package. Journal of Fluency Disorders 11: 93–103.

Ladouceur R, Caron C and Caron G (1989). Stuttering severity and treatment outcome. Journal of Behaviour Therapy and Experimental Psychiatry 20(1): 49–56.

Lefcourt HM (1976). Locus of Control, Current Trends: Theory and Research. Englewood Cliffs, NJ: Prentice-Hall.

Levy C (1987). Stuttering Therapies: Practical Approaches.Beckenham: Croom Helm.

Ludlow CL and Braun A (1993). Research evaluating the use of neuropharmacological agents for treating stuttering: Possibilities and problems. Journal of Fluency Disorders 18: 169–182.

Metz DE, Onufrak J and Ogburn R (1979). An acoustical analysis of stutterers speech prior to and at the termination of therapy. Journal of Fluency Disorders 4: 249–254.

Metz DE, Samar VJ and Sacco PR (1983). Acoustic analysis of stutterers fluent speech before and after therapy. Journal of Speech and Hearing Research 26: 531–536.

Neilson MD and Neilson P (1987). Speech motor control and stuttering: A computational model of adaptive sensory-motor processing. Speech Communication 6: 325–333.

Nittrouer S and Cheney C (1984). Operant techniques used in stuttering therapy: A review. Journal of Fluency Disorders 7: 169–190.

Onslow M, Hayes B, Hutchins L and Newman D (1992). A speech naturalness and prolonged speech treatment for stuttering: Further variables and data. Journal of Speech and Hearing Research 35: 274–282.

Pauls D (1990). A review of the evidence for genetic factors in stuttering. In: Cooper J (Ed) Research Needs in Stuttering: Roadblocks and Future Directions. Rockville, MD: ASHA Report No. 18, 34 -38.

Peters TJ and Guitar B (1991). Stuttering: An Integrated Approach to Its Nature and Treatment. Baltimore: MD: Williams and Wilkins.

Rosenfield DR and Nudelman HB (1987). Neuropsychological models of speech dysfluency. In: L Rustin, H Purser and D Rowley (Eds) Progress in The Treatment of Fluency Disorders. London: Taylor & Francis.

Runyan CM, Bell J and Prosek RA (1990). Speech naturalness rating of treated stutterers. Journal of Speech and Hearing Disorders 55: 434–438.

Smith A (1990). Factors in etiology of stuttering. In: Cooper J (Ed) Research Needs in Stuttering: Roadblocks and Future Directions. Rockville, MD: ASHA.

Smith ML and Glass GV (1977). Meta-analysis of psychotherapy outcome studies. American Psychology 32: 752–760.

Starkweather CW (1993). Issues in the efficacy of treatment for fluency disorders. Journal of Fluency Disorders 18: 151–168.

Stewart T (1992). Attitude change and maintenance of fluent speech in adult stammerers. PhD Thesis: University of Leeds.

St Louis KO and Westbrook JB (1987). The effectiveness for stuttering. In: Rustin L, Purser H and Rowley D (Eds) Progress in the Treatment of Fluency Disorders. London: Taylor & Francis.

Van Riper C (1982). The Nature of Stuttering (2nd Edition). Englewood Cliffs, NJ: Prentice Hall.

Waterloo KK, and Gotestam KG (1988). The regulated breathing method for stuttering: An experimental evaluation. Journal of Behaviour Therapy and Experimental Psychiatry 19(1): 11–19.

Yairi E (1993). Epidemiologic and other considerations in treatment efficacy research with preschool age children who stutter. Journal of Fluency Disorders 18: 197–219.

Part Two: Children's Non-fluency/Stammering

The Development of Dysfluency

Stammering usually begins when the speech and language are developing most rapidly (Bloodstein, 1987; Van Riper, 1982). The child is having to learn to control a speech mechanism that is continuously changing in size and shape because it is growing rapidly. The child is not familiar with how to produce all sounds and to move from one sound to another. In addition, there is a burden of trying to select the right word from an immature and developing vocabulary. Between the ages of 2 and 3 years, the average child's vocabulary will leap from about 50 to 250 words; in fact, towards the end of the third year it is possible that the child will be learning between five and seven new words a day (Studdert-Kennedy, 1987). Furthermore, there are the difficulties related to learning grammar and linguistic structure. Starkweather (1989) suggests a model to clarify the possible underlying pressures on fluency as 'demands' versus 'capacities'. Within 'demands' she categorizes environmental features such as parental speaking rate, directive questioning and self-imposed features, for example, the language level required for satisfaction. Within 'capacities' she includes aspects such as maturity of motor control, paralinguistic abilities, linguistic abilities and social maturity. It is not surprising that many children go through a period of dysfluency at this stage when there is an ever increasing demand on linguistic competence and articulatory proficiency (Adams, 1990; Starkweather and Gottwald, 1990). It has been speculated that the increased incidence of stuttering among those with learning disability is related to the slower acquisition of speech and language and the longer learning period that is required, leading to a longer period of pressures on fluency which may become reinforced.

Most authors would concur with these constitutional, developmental and environmental factors which may underlie the change from normal dysfluency to the establishment of stammering. But most children who are dysfluent will only remain so for a period of months and then progress to fluent speech, and those who stammer may well be unaware of their difficulties (Yairi, 1993). This stammer, often termed 'primary stammering' or developmental dysfluency, is perceptually different from normal dysfluency and noticeable as a stammer to the parents and others, but may not progress to established secondary stammering with the concomitant difficulties of awareness, struggle behaviour and avoidance. These different phases can be usefully termed early non-fluency, borderline stammering and confirmed stammering (Stewart and Turnbull, 1995).

Whilst there is considerable speculation regarding the factors affecting the transition from normal non-fluency to stammer or normal fluency, and the prevalence of the transitional state, it has been noticed that dysfluency in children probably relates to the speech and language development of the individual child. There is little or no information on the longitudinal history of dysfluency and this makes it difficult to evaluate the effectiveness of different treatment programmes. One study that has addressed this issue suggests that the information substantially changes the way that we should review stammering treatment in the future.

Yairi and Ambrose (1992) followed up 27 children for 2 years and a further 21 for 12 years. Of these, nine, by chance, received no treatment. All the children were recruited into the study shortly after they began stuttering. Results indicated that there was a marked deceleration over time in the mean frequency of stuttering-like dysfluencies. Data from individual subjects showed considerable variability in the longitudinal development of dysfluency, but most subjects followed the pattern of the group means. Much of the reduction took place during the early stage of the disorder, especially near the end of the first year post-onset. The authors suggest that it is possible to discriminate between those who will recover and those who will have chronic dysfluency approximately 20 months post-onset. In general stuttering in very young children tended to be a short-lived disorder. This conclusion is complemented by the individual data indicating that the extent of recovery may approximate or even surpass the 79% reported by Andrews and Harris (1964). The rapid improvement of complete recovery of so many children, within the first year following onset, should be carefully considered by investigators of early stuttering. Subjects tested beyond that limit may already represent a rather selective sub-group.

Peters and Guitar (1991) suggest that between 50 and 80% of children who have a primary stammer will recover with or without professional treatment. The authors indicate that the factors related to recovery may be sex (females seem to recover more than males), severity of stammer (less severe improving more rapidly), and more rapid linguistic development.

Literature regarding the transition of normal non-fluency to stammering, is poor. For example, in a review of the literature on stammering from 1967 to 1977, Sommers *et al.* (1979) found that subjects 15 years and younger comprised only 20% of all those who were studied and 5-year-olds and younger accounted for only 3% of the research literature. An exhaustive bibliography of clinical, experimental and theoretical publications referring to children between the ages of 5 and 12 years and for under 5 years (Silverman, 1979) listed 695 reports. However, this literature search went back as far as the 1890s and many of the reports are cursory and disappointing.

Therapy for Children

Many texts cite two approaches to the treatment of children with stammering. The first is an indirect approach where parents are encouraged to create a fluency-enhancing environment; this aims to improve the child's confidence with language by positively listening, using techniques to improve familiarity with phonology, vocabulary and linguistic structure. To this end, parents are encouraged to speak more slowly, attend to the child's speech when he/she is fluent, be less directive and ask fewer questions.

More direct approaches have incorporated relaxation techniques for children, introduction of slowed speech, direct speech and language therapy programmes to improve receptive and expressive language and phonology, and psychotherapy. There have been far fewer research projects evaluating the effectiveness of these different approaches. An approach combining these emphases according to the presenting stage is advocated by Stewart and Turnbull (1995), who hypothesize that therapy should be linked to the phase of dysfluency. Thus, children with early non-fluency should receive no direct intervention, but parental counselling; borderline stammering would require therapy including some direct work and parental counselling, and children with confirmed stammer should follow a programme including direct and indirect work on speaking rate and attitudes along with parental counselling. These approaches will be hard to evaluate without the background of substantial information on the natural history of the disorder itself.

Many children are referred to speech and language therapy at a time when their speech and language systems are rapidly changing, therefore it is difficult to establish a good baseline prior to treatment in order to compare this with post-treatment results. However, some studies have overcome these problems using single-case design.

One study of four children (two boys, two girls) investigated the effectiveness of parent-administered operant verbal stimulation procedures. The authors took speech samples in a number of different settings for 2 months pre-treatment and compared these with those taken 9 months post-treatment. The outcome was found to be favourable, with a marked reduction in dysfluent behaviour that was maintained. The authors note that by making the parents the primary agents in the therapy, the amount of speech therapist time was greatly reduced and they feel that this was a cost-effective way of treating this problem (Onslow *et al.*, 1990).

A similar approach by Johnson (1980) gives detailed information on how to use parents as the main agent in the treatment of dysfluent children between the ages of 2.5 and 17 years. This paper gives detailed information regarding the treatment programme but less clear information regarding outcome. It is possible to infer from the data presented that the programmes were seen as efficacious.

Another investigation of therapists and parents working together (Budd *et al.*, 1986), reviewed 18 children between 8 and 17 years of age who were trained formally in the use of 'stutter-free speech' whilst parents received instruction in how to reinforce and negotiate procedures. Post-treatment there was a systematic reduction in stuttering for 16 of the children and follow-up checks showed a maintenance of post treatment improvement for 6 months. Parents displayed gains in knowledge of child management principles and improved perception of children's behaviourial adjustment. The authors suggest their findings support the efficacy of a multi-faceted behaviourial approach, which includes parents with therapists in the treatment of children's stuttering.

The relationship between a parent and the influence on stuttering behaviour and speaking rate were studied by Guitar *et al.* (1992). This is an interesting study as most of the papers investigating the use of parents tend to train and involve one parent only. However, this study indicates a difference in the influences of each parent at different points during the child's stuttering behaviour. The first study suggested that the mother's speech rate was the only parental behaviour that predicted the child's stuttering. However, in a follow-up study there was evidence that additional behaviours from the father could predict stuttering. The authors advise that stuttering therapy needs to consider the behaviours of each parent differentially in implementing treatment.

Evaluation of a programme using both direct and indirect methods, along with parental involvement, was examined in a study of four children aged 6–9 years by a multiple baseline technique (Caron and Ladouceur, 1989); the direct component of therapy covered the **gentle contact** of articulation and **improved awareness** of stuttering behaviour by both parents and children. The results showed a significant improvement in fluency, a reduction in stammering behaviour and improved parental attitudes and support. The authors feel that the evidence confirms their hypothesis that a combination of direct and indirect treatment results in a clinically significant reduction of stuttering among children who are dysfluent.

The debate regarding the relative effects of indirect versus direct methods was addressed inconclusively by Ramig and Wallice in 1987.

This study exposed one young child to two sessions of indirect therapy, followed by two sessions of both combined direct and indirect therapy. The authors suggest that there were better results with the combined sessions. However, the issue regarding sequential effects was not addressed. The question regarding the relative benefits of the two approaches and the best timing for using them remains unanswered. The essence of both approaches was combined in a programme called simplified treatment for stuttering children (Wagaman *et al.*, 1993). This treatment includes awareness training, relaxation and airflow, along with social support and parental training. The authors examined eight children aged between 6 and 10 years, who had been treated in this way in their homes. They used a multiple baseline technique and found that all children reached the criterion level of less than 3% words stuttered. Furthermore, the reduction in dysfluency generalized to the school setting and was maintained at a post-treatment check, which was held 10–13 months later.

Developing more structured treatment programmes for hard-pressed clinics or busy schools has attracted some attention. Runyan and Runyan (1986) developed an approach called Fluency Rules Therapy Programme in order to assist them to provide therapy, in school, in which a child was allocated two 30 minute sessions per week. The fluency programme incorporated speaking slowly, the use of speech breathing, light articulation contact points, easy speech, prolonging sounds, soft voicing, and reduction in repeating. Nine children aged between 4 years 6 months and 7 years 1 month were studied. Four of these had a less severe stammer at the start of the study. The children's speaking rates and the frequency of words stuttered demonstrated that fluency was improved. This was not due to a reduction in verbal output. In addition, the severity of the remaining blocks was minimal.

There are many substantial challenges remaining in the area of children with fluency disorders. The first is the relationship between predictive factors and outcome. It is critical to establish whether certain factors are indicative of which children are going to develop a more confirmed stammer and which are likely to be more resistant to treatment. A study by Starkweather and Gottwald (1993) aimed to identify the relationship between variables measured at the outset and the termination of treatment. Eighteen families were included in the study and the measures identified as being of interest were:

1. Waiting period between identification of 'a problem' and the onset of treatment.
2. The child's age.
3. Articulatory rate of parents and child.
4. The number of questions asked by parents.

5. Number of interruption of child by parents.
6. The child's percentage of discontinuous speech time.

Relationships were observed suggesting the importance of beginning treatment for stuttering as soon as possible and the possibility of a pattern of negative parental reaction to discontinuous speech in children.

Conclusion

Although there is a general consensus regarding the features of normal non-fluency and those of stammering along with agreed, though not confirmed, hypotheses relating to the underlying causes, there is a noticeable lack of information on the natural course of fluency and the efficacy of preventative speech and language therapy for this client group. Many speech and language therapists intervene with indirect techniques at an early stage of non-fluency but little work has been done to establish whether these programmes are beneficial. Work in this particular field is hampered by having such limited information on the natural course of the disorder itself, making it difficult to evaluate therapy programmes of older children and targeting resources appropriately.

The next challenge for evaluation of the efficacy of stammering for children is to identify the specific aspects of treatment which are effective and lead to improved use of speech (Conture and Guitar 1993). Not surprisingly, most approaches are eclectic and it would be helpful to eliminate those aspects of treatment that are inert or possibly harmful. Interestingly, the aspect that therapy may do harm as well as good is not attended to in the literature and few studies have sought to answer this question.

'Research and clinical experience with stuttering indicate that it is a complex, multidimensional problem' (Gregory, 1973).

References

Adams MR (1990). The demands and capacities model 1. Journal of Fluency Disorders 15: 135–141.

Andrews G and Harris M (1964). The Syndrome of Stuttering. London: Heinemann.

Bloodstein O (1987). A Handbook on Stuttering. Chicago: National Easter Seals Society.

Budd KS, Madison LS, Itzkowitz JS, George CH and Price HA (1986). Parents and therapists as allies in behaviourial treatment of children's stuttering. Behaviour Therapy 17: 538–553.

Caron C and Ladouceur R (1989). Multi-dimensional behaviourial treatment for child stutterers. Behaviour Modification 13(2): 206–215.

Conture E and Guitar B (1993). Evaluating efficacy of treatment of stuttering: School age children. Journal of Fluency Disorders 18: 253–287.

Gregory H (1973). Stuttering: Differential Evaluation and Therapy. New York: Bobbs-Merrill Company Inc.

Guitar B, Schaefer HK, Donahue-Kilburg G and Bond L (1992). Parent verbal interactions and speech rate: A case study in stuttering. Journal of Speech and Hearing Research 35: 742–754.

Johnson LJ (1980). Facilitating parental involvement in therapy of the dysfluent child. Seminars in Speech, Language and Hearing 1(4): 301–309.

Onslow M, Costa L and Rue S (1990). Direct early intervention with stuttering: Some preliminary data. Journal of Speech and Hearing Disorders 55: 405–416.

Peters TJ and Guitar B (1991). Stuttering: An integrated approach to its nature and treatments. Baltimore, MD: Williams and Wilkins.

Ramig PR and Wallice ML (1987). Indirect and combined direct-indirect therapy in a dysfluent child. Journal of Fluency Disorders 12: 41–49.

Runyan CM and Runyan SE (1986). A fluency rules therapy programme for young children in public schools. Language, Speech and Hearing Services in Schools 17: 276–284.

Silverman FH (1979). Bibliography of literature pertaining to the onset, development and treatment of stuttering during pre-school years. Journal of Fluency Disorders 4: 171–203.

Sommers RK, Bobkoff-Levanthal K, Applegate JA and Square PA (1979). A critical review of a recent decade of stuttering research. Journal of Fluency Disorders 4: 223–237.

Starkweather CW (1989). Current trends in therapy for stuttering children and suggestions for future research. In: Cooper J (Ed) Report of NIH Workshop on Trends in Stuttering Research. ASHA Report Number 18.

Starkweather CW and Gottwald SR (1990). The demands and capacities model II. Journal of Fluency Disorders 15: 143–145.

Starkweather CW and Gottwald SR (1993). A pilot study of relations among specific measures obtained at intake and discharge in a programme of prevention and early intervention of stuttering. American Journal of Speech Language Pathology 2: 51–58.

Stewart T and Turnbull C (1995) Working with Dysfluent Children. Bicester: Winslow.

Studdert-Kennedy M (1987). The phoneme as a perceptuomotor structure. In: Allport A, McKay D, Prinz W and Scheerer E (Eds) Language Perception and Production. London: Academic Press.

Van Riper C (1982). The Nature of Stuttering (2nd Edition). Englewood Cliffs: Prentice Hall.

Wagaman JR, Miltenberger RG and Arndorfer RE (1993). Analysis of a simplified treatment for stuttering in children. Journal of Applied Behaviour Analysis 26(1): 53–61.

Yairi E (1993). Epidemiologic and other considerations in treatment efficacy research with pre-school age children who stutter. Journal of Fluency Disorders 18: 197–219.

Yairi E and Ambrose N (1992). A longitudinal study of stuttering in children: A preliminary report. Journal of Speech and Hearing Research 35: 755–760.

Chapter 9
Voice Disorders

Introduction

There is no definition of normal voice. An abnormal voice is one where the quality, pitch, loudness or flexibility are interpreted as being unpleasant or inappropriate to the age or sex of the speaker. For the purposes of this chapter, voice disorder refers to those difficulties arising from disturbance or loss of laryngeal function. It does not include disorders of resonance alone, which are considered with the condition causing the disorder, e.g. cleft palate, dysarthria. Laryngectomy is considered elsewhere.

Estimates of the prevalence of voice disorder, in the general population, are likely to vary depending on the criteria used. Enderby and Phillipp (1986) suggests that the annual incidence of dysphonia in England could be 28 per 100 000 population, basing this calculation on five years of referrals for dysphonia to one general hospital. Recent figures suggest that the incidence in some parts of the United Kingdom is higher. Gordon gives the figure of 89 per 100 000 referrals for dysphonia annually in Glasgow (personal communication, 1994).

Boone (1983) suggests that for phonation disorders in the USA, the prevalence is probably about 3%. La Guait (1972) found that 7.2% of males and 5% of females, out of his sample of 428 adult patients, had voice disorders. Wilson (1979) estimated that 5–6% of the school population in North America had voice disorders. There are no reports of the incidence of voice disorders in a general population.

Voice disorders may be classified as organic or non-organic. Organic disorders may be caused by disease, congenital disorders, malformations, or injury. Another group of organic disorders are the hyperfunctional disorders where misuse or abuse of the voice results in vocal nodules, contact ulcers, or inflammation. Non-organic disorders include functional disorders, which are those unaccompanied by any laryngeal pathology and psychogenic disorders such as hysterical aphonia and dysphonia. Aronson (1980) groups the hyperfunctional disorders and the functional disorders together as being psychogenic disorders caused by stress and tension.

The aetiology of the disorder known as spasmodic or spastic dysphonia is unknown. Hillman *et al.* (1990) claim that evidence is mounting that some of the manifestations are associated with neuropathology. It has been suggested that the symptoms and signs of spasmodic dysphonia might arise from different causes and that the disorder might not be one but several conditions (Aronson, 1980).

Diagnostic Assessment of Voice

Voice evaluation should include a history of the voice disorder, including details of previous voice disorders, the onset of the current voice disorder and its course, and events associated with the onset (Aronson, 1980). Information is obtained on the patient's health, social history, life style, work and stress factors (Colton and Casper, 1990). Boone (1983) and Colton and Casper (1990) stress the importance of the skills of interviewing and counselling in the process of case-history taking in this area where emotional factors are so important.

Recording is made of the patient's voice in a variety of vocal tasks including examinations of respiration, phonation, pitch and resonance. A rating scale may be helpful in quantifying the clinician's impression.

There have been recent advances in the use of methods of recording for the purposes of assessment and treatment of voice disorders. Techniques such as flexible fibre-optic laryngoscopy, allow the larynx to be viewed more effectively with less inconvenience than older techniques (Colton and Casper, 1990) and with the use of video, can provide accessible information and documentation to the patient and professionals (Metson and Rauch, 1992). Electro-laryngography (Abberton *et al.*,1989; Baken, 1992) can give information about the action of the vocal folds without the need for invasive procedures.

Efforts have continued to match improvements in voice subjectively experienced by clinicians or patients following voice therapy with objective measures of various kinds. Davis (1979) describes acoustic measures that have been used and could be further developed to assist in the diagnosis of and screening for voice disorders. Cooper (1974) undertook a spectrographic analysis to compare fundamental frequencies before and after voice therapy for a wide range of functional and organic dysphonias. After successful voice therapy, the individual mean fundamental frequency was higher for 150 out of 155 patients and the author concludes that the use of too low a pitch is a major factor contributing to most types of dysphonia. Fex *et al.* (1994) performed an acoustic analysis on 10 patients before and after voice therapy and found pitch perturbation quotient, amplitude perturbation quotient, normalized noise energy from 1 to 4 kHz and fundamental frequency showed significant change. Schneider (1993) undertook seven sets of acoustic measures at intervals over 2 years with one patient with vocal fold nodules. It was found that the acoustic measurements of mean fundamental frequency, fundamental frequency range and jitter did not relate to measures of clinical change but there was a relationship between vocal fold condition, perceived changes in voice quality and patients' symptoms. Kitzing and Akerlund (1993) analysed tape recordings of 174 voice patients, before and after successful voice therapy, by means of long-time average spectrograms (LTAS). Voice change following therapy perceptually rated as 'considerable' related to significant increase in voice intensity as shown by the LTAS. The authors maintain that individuals in the study showed other changes in LTAS following therapy and suggest that individual LTAS may be used to sharpen perceptual evaluations of voice quality and develop a more precise terminology for these evaluations.

It seems likely that the development of digital computer recording of voice will provide the clinician with easily understandable material to aid diagnosis and record treatment improvements. Airainer and Klingholtz (1993) describe a way in which phonetograms–records of the loudness of the voice at different fundamental frequencies–may be subjected to computer-aided processing to assist in the classification of different types of functional dysphonia.

Gordon (1992) describes the use of airflow measurement during respiration and phonation, recorded by means of a pneumotachograph linked to a computer, to aid in the assessment and diagnosis of some dysphonic patients, to plan treatment and to record progress during treatment. The author claims that this offers an objective record of the effects of treatment that is non-invasive, reliable and simple to use in a clinical setting.

The increased use of diagnostic techniques such as these has been of great assistance in providing more objective measures of the voice, before and after treatment or therapy. However, clinical evaluation of the voice will remain a powerful indicator of the degree of voice disorder.

Medical and Surgical Treatments for Voice Disorders

Recurrent laryngeal nerve paralysis resulting in paralysis of the vocal fold may be corrected by surgery which will enable the paralysed vocal fold to reach the mid-line and make contact with the other vocal fold to reduce the amount of inappropriate voiceless air escape.

Dedo, Urrea and Lawson (1973) undertook a retrospective review of 135 patients who had received a Teflon injection for dysphonia associated with paralysed vocal cord, laryngeal scarring or bowed mobile vocal cord, between 1967 and 1973. The voice had been rated on a five point scale:

1. Paralytic falsetto
2. Whisper voice
3. Severe breathy phonatory
4. Mild-to-moderate breathy phonatory
5. Normal phonatory

One hundred and ten patients (81%) recovered normal voice after Teflon injection, 129 patients (96%) improved at least one category, with particularly good results for patients with laryngeal nerve paralysis only and no scarring or tissue loss due to trauma. The authors comment that the post-injection voice was not always identical to the previously normal voice. Although this study reviews patients up to 5 years after injection, no details are given on the period of time after operation for the above results and the longer term effects remain in question following this study.

Nakayama, Ford and Bless (1993) describe the difficulties of 28 patients with poor results following Teflon injection for glottal insufficiency, using both objective and subjective methods of assessment. The authors conclude that most of the patients studied had been injected poorly, either in the wrong place, or with too much material, or both. Six of the patients in this study had had no vocal fold paralysis at the time of the original Teflon injection and were operated on because of scarred vocal folds (three patients), vocal fold atrophy (two patients), or laryngeal trauma (one patient). Improvement was brought about in some individuals by removal of the implant or with collagen injection. The worst results, following intervention for the problems resulting from Teflon injection, were obtained from two of the six patients whom the authors considered should never have been injected with Teflon.

Tsuzuki *et al.* (1991) describe the results of injecting liquid or solid silicone into the vocal fold in 51 patients with recurrent laryngeal nerve paralysis. They found liquid silicone and solid silicone both effective in improving voice, as assessed by mean phonation time, compared with no treatment. Follow-ups between 4 and 17 years after injection led the authors to conclude that the liquid implant is, ultimately, absorbed and therefore is most useful for temporary voice improvement when the long-term outcome is not known and that solid silicone is most useful in cases where there would be no recovery of vocal fold function.

Polyps can be treated surgically by removing excessive mass from the vocal fold. Frequently small polyps are treated by surgery if they have not responded to voice therapy. It is suggested that, large and old polyps should be treated by surgery, followed by voice therapy (Colton and Casper, 1990). Surgery is recommended for polypoid degeneration of the vocal folds or Reinke's oedema (Boone, 1983; Colton and Casper, 1990). Increasingly, surgery is carried out using lasers.

Matsuo, Kamimura and Hirano (1983) undertook a retrospective review of 191 patients with polypoid vocal folds; 114 patients underwent surgical treatment and data was available for 107 of them. Forty-three per cent recovered normal voice, 48% showed improvement and 9% showed no improvement following surgery. Seventy-seven patients had no surgery. Of 41 patients not referred for surgery, because of the slightness of the lesion, 19 were treated with conservative treatment, such as anti-inflammatory medication, 5 who were not treated did not improve and 17 were lost to follow-up. In six patients where surgery was recommended but did not take place, four people improved after conservative treatment. Assessment was described as taking place by means of follow-up examinations or questionnaires, at least 5 months after treatment, but no further details were given. Speech and language therapy was not mentioned.

In the condition termed 'spastic dysphonia', the vocal folds are tight and tense, resisting airflow. One treatment for this condition has been treated by sectioning of the recurrent laryngeal nerve. Dedo and Behlau (1991) reviewed the results of the current laryngeal nerve section for spastic dysphonia in 300 patients. They found that 82% of patients had no recurrence between 5 and 14 years after operation, 15% had mild-to-moderate recurrence 6–24 months after operation. The voice resulting from this procedure is not normal and may be quiet and breathy. Twelve patients in the study undertook a Teflon injection to correct the breathy voice, but Dedo and Behlau caution that this procedure risks a return to spasticity as the paralysed vocal fold returns close enough to the midline to close the gap. Twenty-eight patients had laser vocal cord thinning to reduce or eliminate recurring spasticity.

Though Dedo and Behlau maintain that recurrent laryngeal nerve section produces a 'permanent cure' for the spasticity of spastic dysphonia, the use of injections of botulinum toxin have become increasingly used for the adductor form of spastic dysphonia (Adams *et al.*, 1993; Blitzer *et al.*, 1988; Kobayashi *et al.*, 1993; Truong *et al.*, 1991; Zwirner *et al.*, 1992).

All describe this treatment, of injection of botulinum toxin into the thyro-arytenoid muscle, as effective. Kobayashi *et al.* (1993) report that an initial effect occurs in the first 24 hours and reaches its optimum level after 4 days. Treatments last for 3–4 months. The quantities of the drug used vary. Adams *et al.* (1993) claim better and longer lasting results with unilateral injections. Kobayashi *et al.* suggests that unilateral injection may prevent diffusion of toxin into surrounding muscles.

Blitzer *et al.* (1992) described the treatment of 32 subjects with abductor spastic dysphonia, by injection of botulinum toxin into the posterior crico-arytenoid muscles. The effect of this operation on voice was measured by subjective ratings. The authors claim that most patients improved to a level of 70% of normal voice. Patients who had more extensive dystonia, tremor or respiratory involvement, did less well. There is no information in these studies about general side-effects or the possible long-term effects of treatment with botulinum toxin injections.

Research into medical and surgical treatments of organic voice disorders have tended to view the treatment in isolation. Whilst in practice most patients receiving such treatment would also be receiving speech and language therapy, this is rarely detailed and the contribution of therapy has not been evaluated. Additionally, many of the measurements in the above studies can be criticized as being unspecific and somewhat crude.

Speech and Language Therapy for Voice Disorders

Hillman *et al.* (1990), describes strategies that may be used alone or in combination. The voice therapist aims to correct faulty functions, to compensate for deficit and to modify the care and use of the vocal mechanism.

A number of general techniques can be applied in the treatment of voice disorders. Relaxation is used to reduce laryngeal tension by means of whole body relaxation, or relaxation exercises to the laryngeal area (Aronson, 1980). Breathing exercises are employed to instruct the patient in the best techniques of breathing for the purposes of supporting voice. Voice exercises of various kinds are used to promote soft initiation of vocalization rather than hard glottal attack and attention is paid to pitch and speed of speech to ensure that these are appropriate.

Prater (1991) stresses the importance of modelling from the therapist and feed-back so that the patient understands clearly what voice quality is to be aimed for. In addition to these general techniques, specific techniques are suggested for particular voice disorders.

Clinicians and patients believe that voice therapy works (Hillman *et al.*, 1990). There are many accounts of treatment that describe therapy and successful outcomes which have resulted. This use of descriptions of group and individual case studies is useful in suggesting ideas for research into treatment. Most recent studies of voice treatment are of this type.

Therapy for vocal abuse or misuse

Vocal abuse or misuse is a common voice disorder affecting children and adolescents as well as adults. Koufman and Blalock (1991), in their review of functional voice disorders, found that 300 out of 406 patients with functional voice disorders had this diagnosis. In addition to instructing patients in the general principles of voice use, emphasis is placed in treatment, on increasing patients awareness of abusive behaviour, such as screaming and shouting, and aspects of the environment likely to be deleterious to voice, such as noise, smoke and other pollutants, and discussing with patients ideas for manipulating environment and routines so that these can be avoided.

Young people are vulnerable to this type of voice disorder (Andrews, 1991). Burk and Brenner (1991) emphasize the need for listening to young people to find out what they need and expect before planning treatment. Andrews and Summers (1991) stress the importance for adolescents of becoming aware of factors important in their vocal rehabilitation so that any resistance to an authority figure telling them what to do can be overcome and a therapeutic partnership established. They suggest the use of quizzes as a flexible and versatile method of providing knowledge about voice. A structured voice therapy programme for adolescent vocal abusers giving practice in using optimum voice production techniques in noisy environments is described by Saniga and Karlin (1991).

Vocal misuse in professional voice users involving vocal tension, muscle tension, poor breath control and abnormally low pitched voice, may be a discrete syndrome. Koufman and Blalock (1988) claim it resolves readily with voice therapy in the majority of cases.

Roy and Leeper (1993) describe treatment for functional dysphonia in 17 patients who were assessed and managed in a hospital setting over a 2 year period by means of one session employing Aronson's manual laryngeal musculoskeletal tension reduction techniques (Aronson, 1990). Sixteen patients improved in objective measures of frequency perturbation and amplitude perturbation ('jitter' and 'shimmer') following treatment, 14 of these being rated as having near normal voice or only the mildest dysphonic symptoms. Thirteen of the 14 had maintained improvement on a telephone questionnaire a week later. These authors point out that at present the assessment of laryngeal elevation is subjective and speculate that the part played by muscle tension in voice disorders may be extremely variable. Although Aronson advocates this technique for all patients with functional dysphonia, it would be helpful to isolate symptoms of laryngeal tension and elevation, in dysphonic patients, that reduce following successful therapy, to support the theory of tension as a causative factor.

This study is interesting in that it employs only one therapeutic technique in the treatment of functional dysphonia, but limited, as studies investigating specific therapies need a control group in order that any improvements can be ascribed to treatment rather than to changes over time and an alternative treatment group to attempt to distinguish specific from general treatment effects.

Andrews, Warner and Stewart (1986) compared two treatments for hyperfunctional dysphonia, EMG feedback and progressive relaxation. Ten women, with hyperfunctional dysphonia, were assigned to five pairs matched by age and severity of dysphonia. One of each pair received EMG feedback treatment and one was treated by progressive relaxation. Both forms of treatment were carried out in once weekly sessions lasting 45 minutes each. Subjects received between 4 and 15 sessions of treatment. Objective and subjective voice measurements were carried out before and after treatment. Results showed that both groups improved following treatment and that improvements were maintained at a follow-up 3 months later. This study again lacks a control and, because both treatments were found to be equally effective, the issue of whether the results can be ascribed to specific or general effects of treatment remains unresolved.

Kotby *et al.* (1991) treated 28 patients with various voice conditions by means of the accent method of therapy (Smith and Thyme, 1976) which teaches diaphragmatic breathing and coordination of breathing and voice. Therapy was administered for 20 minute sessions three times a week, with evaluations after 10 and after 20 sessions of therapy. Twenty-four of the patients showed an improvement on author's subjective and auditory assessment and there were some changes in objective measures. Insufficient subject details were presented to know which patients, or disorders, would be likely to respond best to the treatment.

Behlau, Pontes and Tosi (1991) describe treatment of 10 people, with an average age of 73, using techniques of improving vocal quality with the use of feedback, improvement of articulation and dealing with environmental factors. The treatment was claimed to be successful showing an improvement both in objective measures and in patient satisfaction with voice.

It is suggested that patients with more severe personal problems take longer to respond to therapy for functional voice disorders (Schalen and Andersson, 1992). Some patients respond to techniques additional to speech therapy. Horsley (1982) described the treatment of one woman with psychogenic dysphonia. Hypnosis was introduced after 12 sessions of conventional voice therapy had failed. The author claimed that hypnosis induced relaxation and influenced attitudes in two sessions. Five speech pathologists rated the voice as improved after treatment and the improvement was maintained at follow-up 16 months later. Butcher *et al.* (1987) claimed that, out of 12 patients, unresponsive to speech therapy, six improved both in voice and psychosocial adjustment, following a combined approach using cognitive-behaviourial therapy with speech therapy.

Therapy for hysterical aphonia/dysphonia

Aronson (1980) and Stemple (1993) see the condition as a conversion symptom of an unconscious underlying problem and stress the importance of the patient's readiness to relinquish the symptom in order for treatment to be successful. Boone (1983) says that in this condition, for which he prefers the term 'functional aphonia', the aphonic behaviour is maintained by the reactions of other people and the patient's becoming accustomed to relating to people without voice, that is developing a 'no voice set'. Boone says that it is the clinician's role to find the patient's lost 'set' for voice and the condition has an excellent prognosis.

Specific techniques are recommended for the treatment of hysterical aphonia, e.g. the use of white noise to remove auditory feedback while doing exercises based on coughing and sighing, where voice can be achieved, to recover voice in speech (Prater, 1991). An important aspect of treatment is convincing the patient that the voice can be recovered.

Less usual therapies

In recent years, voice therapists have become involved in the treatment of trans-sexuals, aiming to change physical characteristics such as pitch and also working on stress, timing, inflection and choice and use of words, which may be as important as physical characteristics (Colton and Casper, 1990).

Mount and Salmon (1988) describe the treatment of a 63-year-old male to female trans-sexual who complained of low pitched voice. Treatment consisted of training high pitched levels and appropriate inflection patterns at high pitch, modifying tongue carriage and promoting breathy attack. The patient was encouraged to match her voice contours to that of the clinician by means of the Visipitch. Treatment took 88 one hour sessions over 11 months. The patient achieved a fundamental frequency of voice comparable to that of females after 4 months, but was not perceived as a female on the telephone until after 10 months of therapy. The voice remained satisfactory at a 5-year follow-up.

Blager, Gay and Wood (1988) describe the treatment of four patients with habit cough by use of direct voice therapy work on breathing, relaxation and modification of the cough, together with psychotherapy of various kinds. The authors claim that cough symptoms even of long standing can be effectively reduced by this treatment but acknowledge that further work is needed to determine which combination of treatments are effective for which patients.

Voice therapy is typically undertaken individually. Morris (1992), describing a programme of group treatment for six women with hyperfunctional voice disorder, covering information about voice, stress management, relaxation and practical problem solving, concluded that group treatment is effective in providing help and support for members and is a cost effective way of delivering therapy.

Ranford (1982) gives an account of the treatment of a woman with dysphonia resulting from tension and anxiety. The treatment consisted of auditory monitoring, awareness and correction of tension, optimum use of resonating cavities, use of appropriate pitch level and correct use of residual air. Treatment was carried out twice weekly for 3 months, then weekly, then monthly for a total of 9 months, after which the voice was improved and the patient was happy to be discharged. Assessment by means of xero-radiography and electro laryngography was carried out before and after treatment. Changes in the position of the vocal folds and vocal fold contact were shown following treatment.

Yamaguchi et al. (1993) described a programme of voice therapy for 29 patients with glottal insufficiency. Seventeen patients had vocal fold paralysis and 12 had sulcus vocalis. Therapy was based on pushing exercises to increase vocal fold adduction. Instrumentation measures–an audio recording for both perceptual and acoustic analysis, a strobo-scopic examination and phono-laryngograph to provide measures of flow rate intensity and fundamental frequency–were used to select patients suitable for this type of treatment and were taken at 4 week intervals to provide monitoring and new aims for treatment. Feed-back of targets during therapy was provided with the Visipitch.

The authors found that treatment results for patients with sulcus vocalis were poor but claim the treatment to be efficacious in selected cases, usually in combination with surgery for unilateral vocal fold paralysis. They warn of the dangers of over compensation resulting in hyperfunction.

Evaluation of Voice Therapy

Reviews of patient records and questionnaires

Reviews of patient records and retrospective questionnaires are used in evaluating voice therapy for various types of voice disorder.

Harris and Richards (1992) undertook a retrospective review of functional aphonia in 14 young people, 12 females and 2 males, with an average age of 12.6 years, by means of a questionnaire to speech therapists. All patients were considered cured by patient therapist and ENT Consultant, the duration of treatment varying from one session to a maximum of 12 months. Seven of the subjects' voices returned to normal gradually. Three made a gradual improvement at first, then suddenly achieved normal voice. Four achieved normal voice suddenly and totally.

Lancer et al. (1988) used a retrospective questionnaire to assess the outcome of three types of treatment for vocal cord nodules. Findings seem to indicate that speech therapy, with or without surgery, had a beneficial affect on outcome. There are limitations on the validity of studies of this kind because of the inevitably subjective nature of a retrospective questionnaire. In addition, the sample was small, 20 subjects, and there was a high incidence of smokers in the surgery only group, which may have contributed to the less satisfactory results for surgery alone.

Bridger and Epstein (1983) used retrospective examination of patients' notes to assess treatment outcomes in a review of 109 patients with functional voice disorders and found that, in 56% of cases, the voice was cured – that is, it returned to its pre-morbid state – following speech therapy and in 26% the voice was 'improved' after therapy.

Experimental studies

Neither accounts of successful treatment, whether individual or groups of people, nor retrospective outcome studies, can on their own offer evidence of therapy efficacy. This can only be provided by controlled experimental studies.

Allen, Bernstein and Chait (1991), used a single case study design to describe the treatment of a 9-year-old boy, with a 5 year history of hyperfunctional dysphonia who had failed to respond to 3 years of traditional voice therapy and had developed vocal nodules. He undertook EMG biofeedback training for twice-weekly 30 minute sessions. The subject was encouraged to attempt to reduce muscle tension around the vocal folds. EMG activity levels were stable or increasing at baseline, but following the start of treatment decreased step wise in two conditions, resting and speaking. Voice quality was assessed as severely impaired at baseline and near normal at follow up, 3 months and 6 months later. The nodules decreased in size throughout treatment and were gone at 6 month follow-up.

Single case studies of this type offer evidence that treatment has been effective with one particular individual. Experimental group studies compare the effects of treatment with non-treatment in groups of patients and offers the strongest evidence of whether a particular type of therapy may be successful with a number of patients with the same disorder. The only recent study of this type is that of Carding and Horsley (1992), who found evidence to support the effectiveness of both direct and indirect therapy in the treatment of non-organic dysphonia. Thirty patients were randomly assigned to one of three groups, no treatment, indirect treatment and direct treatment, over a period of 8 weeks. The indirect treatment method included counselling, reassurance and information on vocal hygiene. The direct programme consisted of work on voice, including pitch, loudness, glottal attack, breathing and specific relaxation. Treatments for both direct and indirect therapy was selected from a range of treatments.

Significant improvement in both objective and subjective assessment of voice occurred in the treatment groups compared with the non-treatment group. Nine out of ten patients in the direct treatment and six out of ten patients in the indirect group returned to normal voice function. One patient in the control group showed improvement without any intervention.

The clinician chose from a selection of activities for each treatment condition, making it impossible to be sure which particular treatments might have been effective with each individual. Although the lists of activities given were different for each treatment condition, in the two cases given as examples of each type of therapy, both treatment conditions included a description of the voice problem and how the patients voice production deviated from the norm.

Qualitative descriptions of the subjects indicated that the clinician had opinions about the unsuitability of indirect therapy in particular cases and it is possible that the clinician's beliefs may have affected the outcome of treatment.

The outcome of this study, significant success for the treatment groups, with a rationale for any treatment failures and alternative strategies, offers good evidence that voice therapy is successful in treating this group of patients.

Conclusion

A large gap in our present knowledge relates to the lack of data on the prevalence of voice disorders in adults or in children in the United Kingdom. There is a need for more information on the natural history of these disorders.

There has been a rapid increase in sophisticated instrumentation used in clinics to assist with the diagnosis and treatment of voice disorders (Hillman *et al.*, 1990). This should open up many new avenues of research in the field as improved objective evaluation may facilitate better selection of treatment for individuals and more accurate monitoring. For example Metson and Rauch (1992) described how, in 5 out of 112 patients examined, the use of video laryngoscopy had a direct effect on the medical care by revealing conditions missed by other investigations.

Perceptual judgement of voice quality remains the most important aspect of clinical evaluation of voice and more work is needed to ensure that perceptual judgements are valid and reliable.

In the field of voice disorders, the efficacy of treatment is less frequently questioned because clinicians feel their work to be effective. People with voice disorders often seem to respond quickly to treatment. There is a need for more controlled experimental studies of the treatment of voice disorders. A useful investigation of the efficacy of therapy, would be to compare the frequency and severity of relapse between people who have received speech therapy and those who have not.

The possibility of prevention of voice disorders, in apparently vulnerable groups, such as professional voice users and children, needs to be explored formally.

References

Abberton ERM, Howard DM and Fourcin AJ (1989). Laryngographic assessment of normal voice: A tutorial. Clinical Linguistics and Phonetics 3(3): 281–296.

Adams SG, Hunt EJ, Charles DA and Lang AE (1993). Unilateral versus bilateral botulinum toxin injections in spasmodic dysphonia: Acoustic and perceptual results. Journal of Otolaryngology 22(3): 171–175.

Airainer K and Klingholtz F (1993). Quantitative evaluation of phonetograms in the case of functional dysphonia. Journal of Voice 7(2): 136–141.

Allen KD, Bernstein B and Chait DH (1991). EMG bio-feedback treatment of paediatric hyperfunctional dysphonia. Journal of Behaviour Therapy and Experimental Psychiatry 22(2): 97–101.

Andrews ML (1991). The treatment of adolescents with voice disorders; some clinical perspectives: An introduction. Language Speech and Hearing Services in Schools 22: 156–157.

Andrews ML and Summers AC (1991). The awareness phase of voice therapy: Providing a knowledge base for the adolescent. Language Speech and Hearing Services in Schools 22: 158–162.

Andrews S, Warner J and Stewart R (1986). EMG bio-feedback and relaxation in the treatment of hyperfunctional dysphonia. British Journal of Disorders of Communication 21: 353–369.

Aronson AE (1980). Clinical Voice Disorders: An Inter-Disciplinary Approach. New York: Thieme Stratton.

Aronson A (1990). Clinical Voice Disorders (3rd edn). New York: Thieme Stratton.

Baken RJ (1992). Electroglottography. Journal of Voice 6(2): 98–110.

Behlau MS, Pontes PA and Tosi O (1991). Presbyphonia – treatment of aging vocal deterioration. Acta Phoniatrica Latina 13(3): 275–276.

Blager FB, Gay ML and Wood RP (1988). Voice therapy techniques adapted to treatment of habit cough: A pilot study. Journal of Communication Disorders 21: 393–400.

Blitzer A, Brin MF, Fahn S and Lovelace RE (1988). Clinical and laboratory characteristics of focal laryngeal dystonia: Study of 110 cases. Laryngoscope 98: 636–640.

Blitzer A, Brin MF, Stewart C, Aviv JE and Fahn S (1992). Abductor laryngeal dystonia: A series treated with botulinum toxin. Laryngoscope 102(2): 163–167.

Boone DR (1983) The Voice and Voice Therapy. (3rd Edn). Englewood Cliffs, NJ: Prentice-Hall.

Bridger MWM and Epstein R (1983). Functional voice disorders: A review of 109 patients. Journal of Laryngology and Otology 97: 1145–1148.

Burk KW and Brenner LE (1991). Reducing vocal abuse: 'I've got to be me'. Language Speech and Hearing Services in Schools 22: 173–178.

Butcher P, Elias A, Raven R, Yeatman J and Littlejohns D (1987). Psychogenic voice disorder unresponsive to speech therapy: Psychological characteristics and cognitive behaviour therapy. British Journal of Disorders of Communication 22(1): 81–92.

Carding PN and Horsley IA (1992). An evaluation study of voice therapy in non-organic dysphonia. European Journal of Disorders of Communication 27: 137–158.

Colton RH and Casper JK (1990). Understanding voice problems. A physiological perspective for diagnosis and treatment. Baltimore, MD: Williams and Wilkins.

Cooper M (1974). Spectrographic analysis of fundamental frequency and hoarseness before and after vocal rehabilitation. Journal of Speech and Hearing Disorders 39(3): 286–297.

Davis SB (1979). Acoustic characteristics of normal and pathological voice. In: Speech and Language: Advances in Basic Research and Practice. San Diego, CA: Academic Press.

Dedo HH and Behlau MS (1991). Recurrent laryngeal nerve section for spastic dysphonia: 5-to-14-year preliminary results in the first 300 patients. Annals of Otorhinolaryngology 100: 274–279.

Dedo HH, Urrea RD and Lawson LL (1973). Intracordal injection of Teflon in the treatment of 135 patients with dysphonia. Annals of Otology 82: 661–667.

Enderby P and Phillipp R (1986). Speech and language handicap towards knowing the size of the problem. British Journal of Disorders of Communication 21(2): 151–165.

Fex B, Fex S, Shiromoto O and Hirano M (1994). Acoustic analysis of functional dysphonia: Before and after voice therapy (accent method). Journal of Voice 8(2): 163–167.

Gordon M (1992). Measuring phonation by airflow. Speech Therapy in Practice 6: 6–8.

Gordon M (1994). Personal Communication.

Harris C and Richards C (1992). Functional aphonia in young people. Journal of Laryngology and Otology 106: 610–612.

Hillman RE, Gress CD, Hargrave J, Walsh M and Bunting G (1990). The efficacy of speech-language pathology intervention: Voice Disorders; Seminars in Speech and Language 11(4): 297–309.

Horsley IA (1982). Hypnosis and self hypnosis in the treatment of psychogenic dysphonia: A case report. American Journal of Clinical Hypnosis 24(4): 277–283.

Kitzing P and Akerlund L (1993). Long-time average spectrograms of dysphonic voices before and after therapy. Folia Phoniatrica 45: 53–61.

Kobayashi T, Niimi S, Kumada M, Kosaki H and Hirose H (1993). Botulinum toxin treatment for spasmodic dysphonia. Acta Otolaryngol (Stockh) Suppl 504: 155–157.

Kotby MN, El-Sady SR, Basiouny SE, Abou-Rass YA and Hegazi MA (1991). Efficacy of the accent method of voice therapy. Journal of Voice 5(4): 316–320.

Koufman JA and Blalock PD (1988). Vocal fatigue and dysphonia in the professional voice user: Bogart–Bacall Syndrome. Laryngoscope 98: 493–498.

Koufman JA and Blalock PD (1991). Functional voice disorders. Otolaryngolic Clinic of North America 24(5): 1061–1073.

La Guait JK (1972). Adult voice screening. Journal of Speech and Hearing Disorders 37: 147–151.

Lancer JM, Syder D, Jones AS and Le Boutillier A (1988). The outcome of different management patterns for vocal cord nodules. The Journal of Laryngology and Otology 102: 423–427.

Matsuo K, Kamimura M and Hirano M (1983). Polypoid vocal folds. A 10-year review of 191 patients. Auris Nasus Larynx (Tokyo) 10 (Suppl): S37–S45.

Metson R and Rauch SD (1992). Videolaryngoscopy in the office – a critical evaluation. Otolaryngology – Head and Neck Surgery 106(1): 56–59.

Morris C (1992). Shared problems – shared success. CSLT Bulletin September: 4–5.

Mount KH and Salmon SJ (1988). Changing the vocal characteristics of a post-operative trans-sexual patient: A longitudinal study. Journal of Communication Disorders 21: 229–238.

Nakayama M, Ford CN and Bless DM (1993). Teflon vocal fold augmentation: Failures and management in 28 cases. Otolaryngology – Head and Neck Surgery 109(3): 493–498.

Prater RJ (1991). Voice therapy techniques and applications. Otolaryngologic Clinic of North America 24(5): 1075–1092.

Ranford HJ (1982). 'Larynx-NAD'? CST Bulletin 359 (March): 2.

Roy N and Leeper HA (1993). Effects of the manual laryngeal musculoskeletal tension reduction technique as a treatment for functional voice disorders: Perceptual and acoustic measures. Journal of Voice 7(3): 242–249.

Saniga RD and Karlin MF (1991). Varying signal-to-noise ratios in adolescent voice therapy. Language Speech and Hearing Services in Schools 22: 179–188.

Schalen L and Andersson K (1992). Differential diagnosis and treatment of psychogenic voice disorder. Clinica Otolaryngolia 17: 225–230.

Schneider P (1993). Tracking change in dysphonia: A case study. Journal of Voice 7(2): 179–188.

Smith S and Thyme K (1976). Statistic research on changes in speech due to pedagogic treatment (The Accent Method). Folia Phoniatrica (Basel) 28: 98–103. (Cited in Kotby.)

Stemple JC (1993). Voice Therapy: Clinical Studies. St Louis: Mosby Year Book.

Truong DD, Romtal M, Rolnick M, Aronson AE and Mistura K (1991). Double-blind controlled study of botulinum toxin in adductor spasmodic dysphonia. Laryngoscope 101: 630–634.

Tsuzuki T, Fukuda H, Fujioka T, Takayama E and Kawaida M (1991). Voice prognosis after liquid and solid silicone injection. American Journal of Otolaryngology 12: 165–169.

Wilson K (1979). Voice Problems of Children. (2nd Edition). Baltimore, MD: Williams and Wilkins.

Yamaguchi H, Yotsukura Y, Sata H, Watanabe Y, Hirose H, Kobayashi N and Bless DM (1993). Pushing exercise programme to correct glottal incompetence. Journal of Voice 7(3): 250–256.

Zwirner P, Murry T, Swenson M and Woodson GE (1992). Effects of botulinum toxin therapy in patients with adductor spasmodic dysphonia. Acoustic aerodynamic and videoendoscopic findings. Laryngoscope 102: 400–406.

Chapter 10
Conclusions

Speech and language therapy is frequently viewed as a group of prescribed and precise activities. It is commonly referred to as a single entity similar to a drug as if it is made up of certain precise chemicals required in a certain dose. One of the challenges we face is understanding, describing and detailing the components of therapy in order to evaluate the most active and desirable features, and to eliminate the aspects that are inert or possibly harmful. But this, by itself, may be inadequate as it appears likely that the different approaches by individual therapists are more or less effective with different clients with similar speech/language pathology, but who may have differing personal and psychosocial needs.

There has been interesting debate in speech and language therapy as to whether it constitutes an art or a science, with researchers arguing strongly for one side, or the other. This somewhat sterile debate raises the temperature significantly as values are attributed to one more than the other. For example, in medicine 'science' is traditionally valued more than intuitive or artistic dimensions. The reverse value system may be found in those from the psychosocial disciplines. From the therapists' and patients' viewpoints the value and need for both sides to contribute to healthcare appears essential as it is now acknowledged that health is more than the absence of disease; it also relates to image, quality of life and personal expectations. In some specialities, the scientific area has dominated (dysphasia and cleft palate) whereas in others the intuitive recognition has developed more significantly (stammering). In raising this issue we have inadvertently polarized these aspects and given the impression that psychosocial implications are not scientific; this of course is erroneous but emphasizes the need for improved cross fertilization between specialist areas.

In this literature review it has become evident that researchers rarely look beyond the literature in their own field. For example the present challenges in specialist areas of cleft palate and laryngectomy now include the area of better psychosocial understanding of the related handicap. Research in the area of learning disability and stammering have been addressing these issues for some time and this work could usefully inform across boundaries. However, the fields of learning disability and stammering have major difficulties regarding describing and categorizing sub-cohorts in their populations, whereas other fields have developed approaches that may contribute in developing these.

Research related to speech and language therapy, similar to research by other professions, shows a marked disparity in volume across the specialist areas. Efficacy of therapy for dysphasia has attracted relatively more investment, whereas work evaluating SLT in learning disabilities, and developmental speech and language disorders, has only recently attracted interest and even now the volume and the methodologies used are inadequate for the task. This may be related to the different domains of the clinical practices of these areas. The disorders more closely allied to traditional medical and surgical disciplines were exposed earlier to the philosophy of objective investigation and much of the early work in SLT was fostered by, or associated with, medical research programmes frequently using the related resources and techniques. Difficulties more traditionally associated with education have not had the same stimulus, and objective evaluation has not been seen to be of such value as the development of philosophical and hypotheses description.

Of the NHS resources invested in SLT treatment, the bulk is expended in the area of learning disability and developmental disorders. It appears that the converse is true of research resources and this needs urgent attention.

The concluding remark by Sommers, Logsdon and Wright (1992) is somewhat pessimistic:

> 'It is regrettable that published information in the 1980s was no stronger in meeting these needs (clinical decision making) and in some ways was actually weaker in doing so.'

We do not share their pessimism but realize that there is greater awareness regarding the complexity of addressing some of the issues related to speech and language disorders and these are inhibiting and curtailing research. Greater recognition of the heterogeneity of the groups, and difficulties relating to classification, along with the realization that speech and language therapy is not trying to affect speech, voice, or vocabulary of clients alone, but frequently aims to improve the functioning and psychosocial consequences of the disorders, place significant demands on researchers. The majority of research, in the 1960s, 1970s, and early 1980s, could be conducted unhampered by these sophisticated concerns. More recently, therapists have become aware that research frequently addresses only one aspect of their efforts at intervention and that ways of capturing change in the domains of disability and handicap, along with impairment, are necessary in order to evaluate the effectiveness of their work (Enderby, 1992).

Authors have commented on the difficulty of addressing the general question of 'Does therapy work?' directly. The simplicity of this question belies the answer and is similar to the conundrum posed by asking whether bees talk – the straightforward answer 'Yes' or 'No' would prevent discussion of evidence relating to information on the communication systems of bees, which are now well recognized. Wilson (1993), writing about rehabilitation in general, emphasizes the importance of evaluating specific types of therapy and goals of therapy on specific groups of people. Ideas of education and rehabilitation are based on models of learning and re-education, and the professions involved have as their rationale that people can learn, re-learn and change their behaviour in response to changes in their environment.

Many professionals have become threatened about research and its implications, particularly with the increasing emphasis on changing the patterns of clinical delivery on the basis of research evidence. Studies that have proven effectiveness have often been quoted as supporting treatments beyond those described; research that ended with negative results are often derided for methodological flaws (Siegel, 1987).

Despite the laudable quality and quantity of research underpinning the knowledge base of SLT, many therapists feel threatened and uninformed by research. This may be related to the lack of apparent relevance and poor dissemination of research. Many of the acknowledged difficulties regarding exploiting the value of research in real life situations are experienced by SLTs. Research papers are frequently written in styles difficult for clinicians to understand readily, they may only be available in obscure journals, and they often refer to cohorts of patients of such a purity that they do not form the bulk of a clinical case load. These difficulties along with many others are described by Richardson, Jackson and Sykes (1990). Researchers and those who resource research are encouraged by these authors to take seriously the importance of accessibility of their work if it is to be more than an end in itself.

Priorities for Speech and Language Research

One of the objects of this review was to identify priority areas for research investment relating to the effectiveness of SLT for the major client groups with communication disorders. We describe in the introduction our view that reviewing the efficacy literature alone would not be appropriate as this can only be truly evaluated when the context of the related general knowledge base is considered. Thus, we have also investigated, albeit cursorily, studies and information regarding the underlying pathology, epidemiology, associated difficulties, method of classification and assessment, natural history and prevention. Of course, wherever the literature allowed, we have placed emphasis on the efficacy literature itself. However, this literature has all too often failed in its

aim even before the studies were started, as the objectives of the treatment, the end points and goals, were rarely detailed. We would suggest
that unless there is greater knowledge of therapy aims it is impossible to
ascribe the success or otherwise of any particular method.

Speech and language therapists combine attention to the specific
speech and language disorder (the impairment);[1] along with teaching
the patient/client to improve intelligibility, conversational ability and
general communication (the disability), despite the impairment.
Frequently they use techniques with the client and carers designed to
improve the general standing, autonomy, esteem of the client (the
handicap). Therapy for all client groups therefore aims to improve the
quality of life as well as the specific disorder of the individual, and true
evaluation of the effectiveness of treatment should aim to measure
whether SLT has had an impact on all these areas. There have been no
studies to date which have either disaggregated the components of the
therapy to establish whether treating the impairment, disability or
handicap have been the main aims or had the greatest impact, nor have
there been any studies emphasizing control for these. At present most
studies use measures of impairment even when the therapy may have
been dwelling on psychosocial adjustment. Many patients with speech
and language difficulty have chronic disorders which may not be
'curable'. The role of therapists in improving the patient's quality of life
is as important as evaluating the change of a waveform in those with
more acute conditions.

A summary of our main conclusions identifying research need are in
Appendix II. The comparisons are subjective and relative; there are no
domains that would not benefit from further study, investigation and/or
replication or ratification or should allow complacency. However there
are some pivotal areas that are in urgent need of investment and as yet
have attracted little attention. For example, improved knowledge
regarding the natural course of some disorders is central to treatment
efficacy. Methods of describing disorders, cohorts and identifying subgroups has been attended to in some fields but remains fallow in others.

Whilst there are particular research needs associated with the different client groups there are some common priority areas. The most
apparent of these are:

1. More sensitive outcome measures which can reflect the total impact
   of therapy including psychosocial change.
2. Improved methods of capturing more naturalistic speech language
   samples.
3. Replication of efficacy studies including single case studies to
   strengthen reliability of results.
4. Improved understanding regarding timing and intensity of therapy.

[1]See Appendix I for WHO classification.

5. Studies into the skills required by therapist to achieve desirable outcomes.
6. Methods of describing and disaggregating aspects of therapy.

Acquired dysphasia has stimulated considerable research using a rich mix of methodologies and approaches. However, there is research needed to improve methods of assessing general communicative change in natural settings and in developing a greater understanding of the short- and long-term psychosocial consequences and the related effectiveness of treatment. Improved knowledge relating to the timing and duration of therapy, and the value of long-term support could improve the efficiency of service delivery.

The broad category of children with speech and language disorders will, for this purpose, be linked with the learning difficulties client group as these two groups attract most SLT investment but are the least researched. The need for improved methods of describing and classifying these populations and its many subgroups seems pivotal to much research. Agreement on a core data set to improve access, and comparability of research, along with more detailed retrospective as well as prospective comparative studies, would be valuable.

Research in the area of cleft palate is rich but has mostly addressed surgical management. Different types and intensities of therapy need to be evaluated and small studies need to be replicated. The role of SLT in prevention, as yet, has not been addressed and the psychosocial impact has not been investigated formally.

Given that dysarthria is the most commonly acquired disorder of communication, the amount of related research is disappointing. Most of the SLT research has focused on the difficult area of Parkinson's Disease and less has focused on the other pathologies frequently found in a general case load. Improved methods of detailing the components and goals of therapy is important and again we find that whilst SLT spends considerable time in counselling and long term support of the client group, the psychosocial consequences and the effectiveness of this involvement has not been tested.

The surgical management of laryngectomy has changed radically over the last decade and the related SLT research is impressive; however because of these changes the associated therapy techniques are being reviewed and developed, and require continued investigation. As with the dysarthria client group, the SLT frequently assists with the long-term support and again this involvement should not be exempt from evaluation.

Most of the research into the evaluation of SLT for stammering was generated in the United States of America. There are many indications that practice in the United Kingdom is not identical and thus it is important to conduct properly controlled studies in this country. Improved methods of describing the population to identify the subgroups of pathologies and related difficulties would appear to be essential. It is critical to identify the effectiveness of preventative programmes and to improve the knowledge base related to the natural course of the disorder itself.

There is limited information on the prevalence, underlying pathology and different subgroups of clients suffering from dysphonia. This particular client group calls out for more basic research to identify more accurately the causative agents and factors related to relapse and cure.

Views regarding the value of therapy will change over time. Speech and language therapists work with many different client groups whose disabilities vary in aetiology. They work in various settings, often with other professionals whose own work may influence outcome. It may often be appropriate to plan intervention as part of a team; this may mean the marginalizing or modification of speech and language aims in response to needs perceived by the group as being more important (McGrath and Davis, 1992). Though Siegel (1987) has claimed that it is social and political factors, rather than science, which have an impact on the moral and ethical issues surrounding treatment, some opinions and approaches to ethical matters can be informed by research. A good example of this would be the use of quality-of-life surveys in deciding whether to treat people with progressive conditions.

Does Speech and Language Therapy Work?

Considering the evidence discussed in each of the chapters it would be reasonable to respond with 'Yes' and leave the debate there. However, this would do a dis-service to the professionals and the clients who tackle the complexities of this field on a daily basis. Given the relative youth of this field, the quality and quantity of investigation is laudable. It is easy to deride research conducted a decade or more ago as too simplistic, but each piece of work offers a piece of the jigsaw and assists the selection of another piece to make up the picture. Questions that appeared straightforward 20 years ago now confront the investigator as being more challenging as the details of the panorama becomes better defined.

In some specialist areas most of the jigsaw pieces have been identified. In others only a few pieces have, as yet, been found. In most fields the final picture is challenging and is evolving as we learn not only more about the disorder itself, its relevance, and consequences, but also about the aims and components of therapy.

There appears to be a dichotomy between those advocating qualitative and those advocating quantitative research studies (Enderby, 1992; Minifie, 1989) but both are essential to theory and practice and assist in answering different forms of question. 'The real answer is not to conduct more or less of each type of research but to conduct better research.'

References

Enderby P (1992). Outcome measures in speech therapy: Impairment, disability, handicap and distress. Health Trends 24(2): 61–64.

McGrath JR and Davis AM (1992). Rehabilitation: Where are we going, and how do we get there? Clinical Rehabilitation 6: 225–235.

Minifie F (1989). Research in treatment efficacy: Where is the profession? In: Olswang LB, Thompson CK, Warren SF and Minghetti NJ (Eds) Treatment Efficacy Research in Communication Disorders. Rockville: ASHA.

Richardson A, Jackson C and Sykes W (1990). Taking Research Seriously: means of improving and assessing the use and dissemination of research. London: HMSO.

Siegel GM (1987). The limits of science in communication disorders. Journal of Speech and Hearing Disorders 52: 306–312.

Sommers RK, Logsdon BS and Wright JM (1992). A review and critical analysis of treatment research related to articulation and phonological disorders. Journal of Communication Disorders 25: 3–22.

Wilson BA (1993). Editorial: How do we know that rehabilitation works? Neuropsychological Rehabilitation 3(1): 1–4.

Appendix I

Definition of Impairment, Disability and Handicap

WHO Classification

IMPAIRMENT   Dysfunction resulting from pathological changes in system

DISABILITY   Consequence of impairment in terms of functional performance (disturbance at level of person)

HANDICAP   Disadvantages experienced by the individual as a result of impairment and disabilities. Reflects interaction with and adaptation to the individual's surroundings

Appendix II

Summary of Research Needs

Knowledge related to		Dysphasia	CSLD LD	Cleft palate	Dysarthria	Laryngectomy	Stammer	Dysphonia
Pathology		□	XX	□	□	□	x	x
Associated difficulties		x	□	□	x	x	□	x
Prevalence		□	XX	□	x	x	x	XX
Assessment/ Outcomes	Impairment	□	□	□	□	–	□	□
	Disability	x	x	x	x	x	□	x
	Handicap	x	x	x	x	x	□	x
Natural history		□	XX	□	x	x	XX	x
Prevention		–	XX	x	–	–	XX	XX
Classification		□	XX	□	□	□	XX	x
Therapy Techniques		□	XX	x	x	x	□	□
Efficacy SLT	Impairment	□	XX	□	□	□	□	□
	Disability	XX	XX	XX	□	□	□	□
	Handicap	XX	XX	XX	XX	XX	□	XX

INDEX